550

Adam Jackson is a practising physical therapist and iridologist from London. He runs a private clinic in Hertfordshire and another one in Toronto, Canada. Adam originally trained, qualified and practised Law as a solicitor in England before re-training in natural health care. He studied remedial massage and physical therapy at the Northern Institute of Massage in Blackpool and iridology at the International Institute of Iris-diagnosis in West Germany. He is a member of the Royal Society for the Promotion of Health, the London and Counties Society of Physiologists, and he is founder president of the Canadian Institute of Iridology. He is also the author of *Iridology* in the Optima Alternative Health series.

ALTERNATIVE HEALTH

Massage Therapy

ADAM J. JACKSON

Illustrated by Julie Cannon

DEDICATION

For My Father

An OPTIMA book

Copyright © Adam J. Jackson

The right of Adam J. Jackson to be identified as
author of this work has been asserted by him in accordance
with the Copyright, Designs and Patents Act 1988

First published in 1993 by Optima,
a division of Little, Brown and Company

All rights reserved

No part of this publication may be reproduced,
stored in a retrieval system, or transmitted,
in any form or by any means, without the prior
permission in writing of the publisher, nor be
otherwise circulated in any form of binding or
cover other than that in which it is published and
without a similar condition including this
condition being imposed on the subsequent purchaser.

ISBN 0356 20762 5

Typeset by Leaper & Gard Ltd, Bristol, England
Printed and bound in Great Britain by
Richard Clay Ltd, Bungay

Optima Books
A Division of
Little, Brown and Company (UK) Limited
165 Great Dover Street
London SE1 4YA

CONTENTS

ACKNOWLEDGEMENTS

I would like to thank several people for their help and support in the writing of this book. My dear friend, Mrs Edith Just, who originally guided me into massage therapy. The entire staff at the Northern Institute of Massage with whom I originally trained. Jayne Booth who originally commissioned the book and who subsequently edited it so professionally. Clare Wallis and Hilary Foakes for all their hard work in getting the manuscript into its final form. Mr Ken Woodward, principal of the Northern Institute of Massage, for his help in the research and for writing the foreword of the book. My agent, Sara Menguc, for her continuing help, and last but not least, my wife Karen, for helping to re-type and proof-read the edited manuscript and especially for all her love and support.

FOREWORD

For the past forty years or more, massage has been my life and livelihood. It has served me well in so many ways and, I like to think, so too the many others who have been treated or tutored along the way. My reward is the thought that others now share my dedication and respect for the benefits of the time-tested remedy 'to rub it better'.

Inherent and instinctive in us all, the origin of massage must surely also be that of man himself. Predominant and pioneered as a researched and recognised field of medicine in the nineteenth century, then sadly for the most part, bypassed or abused during the latter part of the twentieth. Thankfully now there are again stalwarts like Adam Jackson who regard massage not merely as a luxury of pampering to those who can afford it, or as little more than an afterthought to physiotherapy, electrotherapy or manipulation, but as a prime therapy in itself. And there are now encouraging signs of the re-introduction and revaluation of massage within the hospital environment.

Therapeutic massage is considerably more than but an element of the now contemporary and rather more charismatic touch therapies such as aromatherapy, acupressure, shiatsu, reflexology and manipulative therapy in its various forms, it is the underlying principle and parent of each. The question remains as to whether it really is the embrocation, liniment, aromatic oil, 'magic sponge' – or fundamentally the adept application of soft-tissue massage that does the trick!

The answer, of course, rests with scientific research, spurred in the first place by the dissemination of knowledge by those with the expertise of technique and the experience of clinical application in the therapy. Any book by such an author will certainly command my attention and interest. More so, as in this particular case, when the author has turned away from a previous sound academic education and qualification within quite a different professional calling towards a training and the subsequent achievement of a successful career in a sphere more dear towards his heart. There is no doubt in my mind that this book is a sound primer which will help guide other feet – and hands! – towards the aptitude of the skilled remedial masseur and the appreciation of the touch of the therapeutic hands.

Hopefully, too, it will initiate the scientific research and clinical tests to prove the therapy beyond any reasonable doubt! Through the Education and Research Development Trust of our mutual professional body, the L.C.S.P. (*see* Appendix), such facility now exists and the advancement of medical science now provides the means hitherto unavailable to the pioneers who instinctively and intuitively understood its worth. This is a book to regenerate the long out-of-print 'classics' on massage penned during the early part of this century.

Massage is much more than mere 'rubbing it better', it is an art, a skill and a science.

Ken Woodward, FLCSP (Phys.)
Principal, the Northern Institute of Massage.

INTRODUCTION

Why another massage book? What makes this one so special? These are the questions several people asked me when I told them I was writing a book on massage therapy. It is indeed a fair question, bearing in mind that there have been countless books written on the subject. But, to this day, most massage books on the bookshelves are still confined to sensual or sexual massage, filled with glossy pages containing pictures of half-naked men and women. By contrast, this book places much greater emphasis on massage as a form of holistic health care.

Massage therapy is a subject about which I feel very strongly because it has given me a very rewarding and worthwhile profession and enabled me to help a great many people over the years. The sad thing is that until fairly recently, it has been largely ridiculed, or even worse ignored by the medical establishment.

Like many people, I had always associated massage more with the pampering of beauty salons and health farms than with natural medicine. When I wanted to embark on a career in a complementary health profession, I couldn't understand why the many health practitioners I asked (including osteopaths, acupuncturists and physiotherapists) came up with the same answer: massage therapy. But I soon came to learn that massage therapy is far more than merely rubbing or stroking various parts of the body. It is the therapeutic manipulation of the soft tissues of the body – the muscles, tendons and ligaments – and has been used for thousands of years to promote health and to help treat a variety of ailments from joint sprains and muscular strains, to headaches, constipation, nervous disorders, and even high blood pressure.

In the succeeding chapters I have drawn on my clinical experience and the available medical and health literature to try to show massage in its true light, as a serious and relevant therapy that will, I believe, once again play an important role in primary health care and the future of medicine.

Adam J. Jackson

1
WHAT IS MASSAGE THERAPY?

Massage should certainly be considered a valuable resource in therapy as well as health promotion. Those who would think otherwise have probably never had a good massage.
                    Dr David Sobel, Chief of Preventive Medicine,
        Kaiser-Permanent Medical Center, San Jose, California.

No one is quite sure from where or when the word 'massage' originated, and there is still confusion as to what it actually means. Most dictionaries suggest that it may have derived from the Greek word *massein* meaning 'to knead' or the arabic word *mas'h* meaning 'to press softly', and then go on to define massage rather vaguely as the 'rubbing and kneading of muscles'. *Taber's Medical Dictionary* describes it as 'Manipulation, methodical pressure, friction, and kneading of the body'. Put very simply, massage is 'the manipulation of the soft tissues of the body – the muscles, tendons and ligaments.'

Massage therapy is the study of specific massage techniques for the promotion of health and the treatment of disease. It is a skill, an art and a science which can only be acquired through study of human anatomy and physiology, together with professional clinical training and, of course, hands-on experience and practice.

The massage therapist's hands are his most important tool through which he not only treats a patient but also detects physical and sometimes emotional problems. Just as a parent will touch a child's forehead to detect a temperature, or feel the child's glands for swellings; so too does the massage therapist palpate the patient's body to determine the condition of the tissues and the likely source of any pain or symptom, and thus the correct type of remedial treatment. A trained massage therapist's fingers become more seeing than his eyes. In massage therapy, the most important things are often invisible to the eyes, and it is only with the fingers that we can 'see' the patient's condition accurately.

There are many different types of massage just as there are many different ways of manipulating tissues whether by kneading whole muscle groups as in Swedish massage or by applying pressure to a specific area or point on the body as in reflexology or shiatsu (acupressure). However, the major part of massage therapy throughout Europe and North America is Swedish massage, the basic techniques of which are described in Chapter 8.

HOW DOES IT WORK?

It is no great mystery why massage therapy is such a successful remedial treatment for many diseases, disorders and deformities. Massage principally works through the various body systems in one of two ways – a mechanical action and a reflex action.

THE MECHANICAL EFFECT OF MASSAGE

A mechanical action is one created by physically moving the muscles and soft tissues of the body. The therapist moves the tissues using pressure and stretching movements, and thereby cleanses them of accumulated acids and deposits. It is the mechanical action that physically breaks up fibrous tissue and loosens stiff joints.

The mechanical action of massage therapy also stimulates circulation by assisting the flow of blood and lymph throughout the body. Tense muscles constrict the blood vessels and inhibit circulation. Relaxing the muscles with massage takes pressure off the arteries and veins and allows the blood to flow more freely. The manipulation of the muscles also squeezes the veins and lymph vessels and literally pushes the blood and lymph fluids through the body.

THE REFLEX EFFECT OF MASSAGE

The best explanation I have heard of a reflex was given by a lecturer during a massage therapy class. He asked the students to imagine that they were on safari and photographing the animals. They were asked to imagine that they had become so enthralled by the beauty of the scenery that they had found themselves separated from the rest of the group. Suddenly, and without warning, as they looked through the camera lens, they found that they were face to face with a lion standing 10 metres away. What would they do?

One student said he would run; 'But the lion will catch you within a few seconds,' the lecturer said. Another student said he would climb a tree; 'Even if there was a tree close enough to where you are standing, the lion would climb up after you', said the lecturer. One by one the students' suggestions were dismissed until one courageous student asked the lecturer, 'Well, what would you do?'

'Simple,' said the lecturer, 'I would bend down, pick up some soft excrement beneath my feet, and throw it into the lion's face. The creature would be so shocked and offended that he would probably run away.'

'But how do you know there will be some soft excrement

directly beneath your feet?' asked the student.

The lecturer replied, 'Because that is a reflex!'

A reflex action is an involuntary response to a specific stimulus. When a doctor asks you to sit with one leg crossed over the other and then lightly thumps a point just below your knee, the chances are that your leg will involuntarily fly up into the air. This is reflex caused through the nerve in the leg having been stimulated.

A reflex is created when treatment of one part of the body affects another part of the body. It is much like pressing a light switch on the wall causes the light bulb in the centre of the room to turn on. Just as the wall switch is connected to the light bulb by a channel of energy called electricity, so too are different parts of the body connected to each other, not just by flesh and bone, but by nerve pathways, blood vessels or, as in Chinese medicine, flows of energy called 'meridians'.

It is for this reason that you can massage your feet and relieve a headache, or that you can massage a person's lower back and alleviate pain in their legs. And it is for this reason that Chinese massage therapists treat a patient's stomach complaint by massaging their arms.

THE FOUR STAGES OF HEALING

In massage therapy, as with most other forms of physical therapy, there are four stages in the healing process: relief, correction, strengthening and then maintenance.

Relief

Massage therapy will first aim to alleviate any pain by sedating the sensory nerves, stimulating blood flow and reducing muscle tension. Cryotherapy (ice therapy) and the opposite heat treatment are both often used to help at this stage. The ice helps to reduce inflammation and the heat assists muscle relaxation and increases blood flow to the area.

The first few treatments will not necessarily eliminate the underlying cause of the problem but they are usually effective in relieving the pain, which is the most important consideration when a person first walks into a clinic.

Correction

Once the pain has been alleviated, the underlying cause of the problem needs to be corrected otherwise the pain will simply return. This will involve rebalancing the muscles, clearing away congested lymph congestion from the tissues and freeing any adhesions (fibres knotted together) or fibrosis (scarring) which may be affecting the tissues. The number of appointments required at this stage will depend upon the state of the injury and the general health of the patient.

Strengthening

After the tissues have been corrected, they should be strengthened to prevent further damage injury. If, for instance, a person has suffered a sprained ankle, the first two stages eliminate the pain and clear the congestion in the tissues. But the ankle joint will usually still be weak at this stage as a result of the trauma of the injury and the length of time it may have been rested. The tissues around the joint will therefore have to be strengthened so that the joint is able to cope with normal activity without the threat of repeated or additional injury.

Maintenance

It is always a good idea to have continuing massage therapy after an injury has been fully treated, particularly when a joint has been injured, because if ligaments have been damaged they will never regain their original strength. This is because the ligament tissues that surround a joint and hold it in place do not contract, and therefore if they are stretched, they will not be able to hold the joint in position as well as they did before the injury.

Maintenance is preventive medicine, helping to keep the tissues healthy and avoid unnecessary injuries in the future. Most people prefer to have regular monthly or bi-monthly treatments to help stay well rather than suffer intermittent injuries that require remedial treatments.

MASSAGE AND ELECTRICAL THERAPIES

The further human society seems to advance with modern technology, the more dependent we are on machinery, and the further we become separated from the human touch. Electrical machines started to become fashionable over 50 years ago and very gradually the science of massage was almost totally dropped by the chartered physiotherapy profession. One of the best used textbooks on physiotherapy is *Tidy's Physiotherapy* which was first published in 1932 under the title *Tidy's Massage and Remedial Exercises**, a title reflecting the import-ance of massage to the physiotherapy profession, a profession which at that time was called The Chartered Society of Massage and Medical Gymnastics. By its eleventh edition in 1986, massage had virtually disappeared from the book's pages.

But history has shown that this change in emphasis in

* The title was changed to *Tidy's Physiotherapy* in the edition published in 1991.

physical medicine did not improve the efficacy of physio-therapy, but rather impaired it. The medical establishment is only now beginning to learn that hands-on therapies cannot be bettered by electrical machinery.

There are, of course, several electrical machines that are very useful in the treatment of many disorders. For instance, the faradic machine sends electrical impulses into the muscles causing contraction of the muscle tissue. This is undoubtedly of enormous benefit to patients who are bedridden or suffering paralysis because it helps to prevent muscle wasting. But in many instances, electro-therapies are over-utilised and mainly used as a matter of convenience. It is far easier, and quicker, for hospital physiotherapists to treat people with machines than for them to be treated individually by massage therapy because a typical massage treatment can take between 30 minutes and an hour.

Many appliances are of dubious therapeutic value too. In physiotherapy colleges, students have been taught that when they come to purchase machinery, they should make sure that it has at least three visible flashing lights. If they had to choose between two machines that did the same job, they should always choose the one that looked more impressive to the patient and this would usually be the one with the most lights. Why? Because there is great value in the patient believing that the treatment works. This is called the placebo effect and has been demonstrated in clinical studies time and time again. If you were to give a sugar tablet to 100 people suffering with the same ailment and tell them that it was a proven cure, whatever their condition 30–40 per cent will get better purely because they believed they would.

An interesting study was carried out at a hospital in Birmingham. The chief physiotherapist had removed the fuse from the diathermy machines because there had been worries about the machines causing burns to the deep muscle tissue. The physiotherapists continued to use the machines without knowing that the machines were not in fact working. Yet after two years, the records showed that nearly 40 per cent of the patients treated still managed to have fully recovered without any other form of treatment.

I once had a discussion with a consultant rheumatologist at King's College Hospital, London, who told me that, as far as he was concerned, ultrasound machines had no therapeutic value. He had carried out studies which revealed that there was no difference whether ultrasound was given or not. He also mentioned that most of the machines he used had not been calibrated properly by the manufacturer and there was therefore no difference in the output when the machines were on high or low.

This is not to say that electro-therapies do not have a place in physical medicine, but their place should not be at the expense of hands-on treatment and care.

It is very sad that the physiotherapy profession continues to exclude massage from its practice. One young physiotherapist who had trained at a teaching hospital in London confessed that out of her three years full-time training, she only received 12 hours of hands-on massage experience. Yet rarely, if ever, can electrical machinery surpass the therapeutic effects of human care and contact. Human touch contains an energy within itself that promotes healing. The power of the human touch and the individual attention of massage therapy can never be replaced by a machine.

THE HEALING TOUCH

'The human touch brings feelings of warmth and being cared for. This greatly increases our sense of well-being.'
Dr Chandra Patel,
The Complete Guide to Stress Management.

Touch itself has healing qualities. Many scriptures speak of the ancient healers laying on of hands to heal the sick. No one really understands the power of touch and what makes it so effective but one interesting study carried out at the Harvard Medical School in Massachusetts has shed some light on the subject. Patients were divided into two groups before similar operations. One group received the standard, fairly cursory briefing by the anaesthetist the night before their operations while the other group were greeted by the doctor who held their hands as he explained in a warm and caring way about their operations. The latter group required fewer drugs and were released from hospital an average of three days before the others.

AN INSTINCTIVE THERAPY

Massage is an instinctive therapy – not just a human instinct, it is used by most of the animal kingdom as well. Watch animals in pain and you will see that they too rub their bodies to ease the pain.

Imagine you are back at your office or other place of work during the day when you begin to feel a throbbing headache. There are no medications available, so what would you do? Most of us instinctively begin to rub around the temples and many of us find that this usually causes the pain to subside. Similarly, gentle rhythmic stroking down the neck of a person suffering anxiety or tension will often induce relaxation and soothe and calm the nervous system.

When you bang your elbow, the first thing you do is rub it and doesn't this alleviate the pain? When children suffer tummy upsets, the first thing they do is hold their tummy and then, pressing down firmly, they make slow, circular movements. Once again the pain is usually alleviated. This is massage therapy – a natural, safe, instinctive and extremely effective hands-on therapy which promotes health and treats many diseases, disorders and deformities.

2
THE HISTORY OF
MASSAGE THERAPY

Massage is, without doubt, the oldest form of physical medicine known to man, traceable to the earliest medical manuscripts. Massage is prescribed in the *Nei Ching*, a compilation of Chinese medicine first written in 400 BC but reputed to be 4000 years old, and therapeutic massage is still taught in the Indian Ayurvedic system of medicine dating back to 1800 BC.

Massage was also advocated by the Greek physician, Hippocrates (known as 'the father of medicine' in the West) who was born in the fifth century BC. He wrote: 'Rubbing can bind a joint that is too loose, and loosen a joint that is too rigid.... Hard rubbing binds, much rubbing causes parts to waste, and moderate rubbing makes them grow'.

It was also widely practised by physicians in Roman times. The Roman Emperors' renowned physician, Galen, wrote at least 16 books relating to massage and exercise, and prescribed massage for the injured gladiators. Another renowned Roman physician, Celcus, treated with massage and recorded that 'chronic pains in the head are relieved by rubbing the head itself'. History also records how Julius Caesar was massaged to relieve neuralgia.

Massage is not only the oldest physical therapy, it is the parent of all other physical therapies including osteopathy, chiropractic, physiotherapy, reflexology and even acupuncture. The ancient Chinese healers were massaging their patients long before they were sticking needles into them. Chiropractic and osteopathic manipulations were all developed by physical therapists who were using massage as a primary treatment. Reflexology, the very popular system of compression massage to the feet, was first developed by a masseuse named Unice Ingham as an adjunct to her massage therapy. The Chartered Society of Physiotherapy in the UK was, less than 100 years ago, known as the Society of Trained Masseuses.

Yet very little is recorded of massage, or indeed any other physical medicine in Europe between the decline of the Roman Empire and the early Middle Ages. The Catholic church had taught that the human body was sinful and it was not until the sixteenth century that medicine slowly began to re-learn much of what had been lost and then to make further progress.

By far the greatest advancement of therapeutic massage recorded in history was made by a Swedish professor, Peter Henrik Ling (1776–1839), who established an institute in Stockholm for the teaching of massage and medical gymnastics. Professor Ling created a scientific system of therapeutic massage known as Swedish massage which was distinguished from the unscientific rubbing employed in Turkish baths*.

Professor Ling's work was rewarded by the Crown and in 1838 a Swedish massage institute was opened in London. In 1877, Dr S.W. Mitchell introduced massage to the USA, and massage institutes were also established in Holland, France

---

*It is sad indeed that some medical writers still, wilfully or through ignorance, state that Swedish massage is a sensual or sexual massage performed by blonde nymphettes. Dr Vernon Coleman, in his book *Natural Pain Control* (Century/Arrow) p. 116, wrote: 'Swedish massage is a phrase used to describe the sort of service usually offered in topless massage parlours. The name is presumably derived from the fact that the Swedes are supposed to enjoy pretty free love lives.'

and Russia. In England, the Northern Institute of Massage was formed in 1924 and still continues to this day to train professional massage therapists.

Towards the end of the nineteenth century, massage had become a science and became a common medical treatment employed in clinics and hospitals, frequently being prescribed by eminent surgeons. However, it was about the same time that 'massage parlours' were being set up as a cover for prostitution. It was to protect the respectability of massage therapy that, in 1894, a group of women in England formed the Society of Trained Masseuses which later became the Chartered Society of Massage and Medical Gymnastics before changing its name again in 1934 to what is today known as the Chartered Society of Physiotherapy. Although the word 'massage' was dropped from its title, massage remained a major form of treatment used by physiotherapists until the introduction of electrical apparatus which became fashionable. Gradually, massage was discarded by the very body of professional people which had been formed to protect it.

But a hard core of people remained who believed in their work and continued to develop the practice of therapeutic massage achieving remarkable success where others had failed. In the UK, the London and Counties Society of Physiologists, formed in 1919, still remains the largest body of professional massage therapists and has served to maintain the standards and codes of practice of the profession and has approximately 2000 practising members. In the USA, massage therapy has grown rapidly; for instance, the American Massage Therapy Association (the oldest professional organisation for massage therapy in America) has grown by more than 500 per cent since 1983, from 1500 practitioners to over 8000.

MASSAGE TODAY

The public image of massage is changing. Only 10 years ago, massage therapists practised mainly at health clubs, in beauty parlours, or made house calls. Today, they work for athletic teams, in high school and college sports programmes, alongside chiropractors and osteopaths, and in hospitals and hospices.

Massage has steadily attracted admirers – among them such notable celebrities as President Bush, Bob Hope, Meryl Streep, Lee Iacocca, as well as sporting personalities such as Australian marathon runner, Robert de Castella, the US long-distance runner, Mary Decker Slaney, Lasse Viren, Joan Benoit and many other top-class athletes. Massage therapy has also been endorsed by numerous national and international sports clubs and sporting associations in the Far East, Europe and North America.

MASSAGE IN THE MEDIA

In the past, massage was only found on the beauty pages of women's magazines. But today massage is featured regularly in scores of publications, and not just the professional journals or health magazines. In the UK, serious newspapers such as the *Sunday Times*, the *Independent*, and the *Guardian* have all carried articles on massage therapy, and in the USA, the *New York Times*, the *Wall Street Journal*, *Forbes*, and many others have all given respectful space to what is arguably the fastest growing health field in complementary medicine.

Replacing negative stereotypes of massage with positive images has been a slow process. *Newsweek* magazine provides a good example. A story in an April 1971 issue focused on thinly disguised houses of prostitution called 'massage parlours' where mostly untrained 'masseuses' performed a variety of rubs. But 13 years later, the magazine reported an entirely different story – that massage had gone mainstream. It was 'no longer associated with pale preludes to sex in sleazy parlours or confined to the get-in-touch-with-your-body crowd of the 70s.' Those who performed on athletic fields, in board-rooms, or on stage now found massage indispensable for staying in shape and achieving their best. And it was the massage therapists they turned to. Then, in 1989 *Newsweek* reported once again the rising popularity of massage, this time in corporate stress management programmes which extended to the US State Department.

How did this turnabout happen? Several trends brought about this change in public attitude: people became more concerned about their health and literally threw themselves into fitness activities. On television we watched massage therapists work magic on runners weary from gruelling marathons, on cyclists during arduous mountain races, on athletes in Olympic stadiums, on football players, weightlifters and gymnasts. The official stamp of respectability came when world class champions expressed their gratitude for massage therapy.

Today massage therapy is without doubt one of the fastest growing forces in the field of health care which is moving beyond the beauty salons and health clubs and into hospitals and clinics, the sports field, the theatre, and even into the offices of commerce and industry.

The experience of the last 50 years has shown that neither drug therapy nor electro-therapies can replace the remedial benefits provided by the trained massage therapist and in very recent years massage has once again begun to be taken seriously. The work of Clare Maxwell-Hudson, a leading masseuse in the UK, has done much to bring the art of massage therapy into the public domain and also into hospitals. Her work in hospitals with cardiologists, surgeons and the nursing staff has demonstrated to the medical profession, at first hand, the value that massage therapy has to offer clinical medicine.

Researchers have begun to undertake comprehensive studies involving massage therapy and have obtained such astounding results that massage therapy is now being given the respect it deserves and is once again being employed in mainstream medicine.

3
MASSAGE IN HEALTH CARE

Massage has an important medical role to play.
                                        Dr Vivian Kriss MD.

In 1987 an article appeared in the *Bradford Telegraph* entitled 'A Medical Role for Massage'. A female medical doctor, Dr Vivian Kriss, believed so strongly in the therapeutic value of massage therapy that she retrained in massage therapy and then gave up her position as a house surgeon at the Bradford Royal Infirmary to work full-time as a massage therapist. 'Massage,' she said, 'has an important medical role to play. It seems to stimulate the circulation, nervous system and muscles. It is a way of enhancing the body's own healing processes.'

In the past, physicians quite naturally adopted massage as the main form of treatment for most muscular and skeletal disorders ranging from simple muscle strains and sprained joints, through to osteo- and rheumatoid arthritis and rheumatism. It was also used very successfully for many spinal deformities including scoliosis (lateral curvature of the spine), spondylitis (inflammation of the spinal cord) and osteoporosis (brittle bone disease). But massage therapy was not just confined to musculo-skeletal conditions; it was also found to help conditions affecting the blood and lymph circulation, the nervous system and was, as a result, prescribed for heart and circulatory disorders, as well as most chronic degenerative diseases including multiple sclerosis, polio, motor neurone disease, brain tumours and even cancer.

In fact, massage was once part of conventional medicine with nurses being trained in massage therapy. Slowly however, the hands-on treatment of massage was discarded in favour of the electro-therapies of machines and group remedial exercises. The Chartered Society of Massage and Medical Gymnastics changed its name in 1934 to the Chartered Society of Physiotherapists. It was from that time that massage gradually ceased to be seen in hospitals in the UK and was neglected by the very body of people established to preserve and promote it.

However, after years of derision and neglect, clinical studies have now proven the benefits of massage. Researchers and doctors are beginning to sit up and take notice of this humble form of treatment. Slowly, but surely, massage is returning to hospitals. From delivery wards and premature baby units to heart units and hospices, massage is being recalled to mainstream medicine.

THE BENEFITS OF MASSAGE THERAPY

Massage affects the body in so many ways, which explains why it is such a versatile therapy and is used to help treat so many different ailments. It improves blood and lymph circulation, disperses oedema fluid (water retention) and helps cleanse the muscles of lactic acid and other body waste by-products. Massage helps breaks down fibrous adhesions (knotted tissues) and relieves muscle spasm, muscle stiffness and soreness. Massage provides general and specific relaxation of the muscles and, in so doing, alleviates physical and emotional tensions as well as pain. It also seems to stimulate the body's immune system and thereby assists physical recovery from acute and chronic ailments.

Last, but not least, massage also helps to relieve pain naturally by encouraging the production of endorphines (natural pain killers) in the body. In fact the benefits of massage therapy seem endless. It has even been shown, in controlled clinical studies, to be an effective aid in the treatment of mental illness including depression and anxiety.

THE BENEFITS OF MASSAGE IN CHILDBIRTH

In 1989 the James Paget Hospital in Great Yarmouth conducted a brief experiment to see whether massage during labour might ease the process of giving birth. Pregnant women were massaged with the relaxing essential oil of lavender during the early stages of contractions, and then with peppermint oil, renowned as a stimulant, as the delivery stage approached. None of the women who participated in the experiment required pethidine or epidurals to relieve the pain of giving birth.

THE BENEFITS OF MASSAGE FOR YOUNG CHILDREN

Massage has also been shown to be effective for infants in hospitals too. Yehudi Gordon, a London obstetrician, states: 'Massage helps reduce colic, constipation, coughs, colds and irritability. It is a very powerful way of communicating non-verbally.'

For instance, in 1990 the *Sunday Times* newspaper carried an article entitled 'Healing touch helps young recover'. Rebecca Colpitts, a nine-year-old girl, could not move her arms or legs or speak when she was taken into the intensive care unit of Guy's Hospital, London. Rebecca had been the victim of a road accident and suffered from a severe head injury and bone fractures. She did not respond to anyone in the hospital until a staff nurse started gently massaging Rebecca's leg that was not in plaster. Moments later Rebecca would visibly relax, and against all expectations, Rebecca soon started talking, nodding and smiling with the help of regular massage.

For children like Rebecca massage is an effective treatment preventing muscle wastage and maintaining adequate circulation to limbs during rehabilitation and apparently speeding physical recovery. It is also evident that the massage therapy brings about noticeable psychological benefits.

Doctors and nurses at the hospital began realising for the first time the psychological benefits of massage brought about by the personal care and communication of hands-on therapy. A neurologist recommended scalp massage instead of drugs for a young child suffering with severe headaches. Such was the success of the treatment that each child on the ward was given their own bottle of aromatherapy massage oil. Orange blossom, lavender, lemon, and camomile were all used and paid for from the ward's budget, but the expense was wholeheartedly approved by the doctors and nurses who could see for themselves the obvious benefits of the scheme.

The staff nurse who introduced the scheme, Ms Trudi Ward, felt that massage could have particular benefits for sick children. 'We have children with serious conditions here – brain tumours, cerebral palsy, severe epilepsy, meningitis, infantile spasm. Babies with infantile spasm (involuntary muscular spasm) and children with cerebral palsy are terribly tense, while brain irritation makes those with meningitis extremely irritable.

'Massage can help by promoting relaxation. It is also diversionary for the children and a nice way of giving personal attention as well as toning the limbs and improving circulation,' she said.

The massage also served to enable nurses to build the trust

and confidence of the children who had previously associated nurses mainly with drugs or needles. One young girl with a brain tumour would scream whenever nurses came near her as she associated them with the nastier things – injections, radiotherapy and pills. It was the massage therapy that broke down her negative associations with the nurses.

Ms Ward said she had not seen one negative response by a child to massage therapy. Even those who cannot talk – the babies, infants with brain damage, cerebral palsy, and the like – give a positive response by unclenching fists, calming down or falling asleep.

FROM THE HOSPITAL TO THE HOME

Young children in hospital often blame their parents for bringing them into hospital and may feel insecure or harbour resentment after a stay. Massage is one way a parent can help break down this type of barrier with a gentle, loving touch. After all, if massage can break down the barriers between nurse and child, it can also help a parent re-establish and communicate care and love for the child.

THE BENEFITS OF MASSAGE FOR MENTAL ILLNESS AND DEPRESSION

There is no doubt that stress may certainly be relieved by massage, and in some cases might be an important adjunct to psychotherapy.

Massage has been shown to help some mentally ill and developmentally retarded children. These children often demonstrate self-injurious behaviour which sometimes results in admission to hospitals or institutions for long-term care. Sometimes drug therapy can do nothing to help these children and, in fact, some drugs are now thought to make them worse. When all other available therapies prove inadequate to control this behaviour, massage always remains helpful.

An interesting case was reported in 1991 in the *Journal of Developmental Medicine and Child Neurology* of a 14-year-old girl with severe self-injurious behaviour who had been treated unsuccessfully for over 10 years before making an astonishing improvement aided by massage therapy.

At the age of three, the little girl had an IQ of 33, her social development level was equivalent to a child of 17 months, and her physical development was that of a child of 24 months. Many drug therapies were offered over the years, but none were in any way useful. One behavioural programme was successful for six weeks, but symptoms then returned.

Finally, an expert on self-injurious behaviour was called in and a recommendation was made for a treatment programme, to include individual attention with massage twice each day. The little girl's behaviour steadily improved after the programme was implemented, especially (it is reported) in response to the massage treatments.

A study conducted by the University of Miami again high-lights the physiological and psychological benefits of massage therapy in caring for the mentally ill. In this study, 52 children and teenagers hospitalised for depression and adjustment disorder were divided into two groups. For five days, one group was given a 30-minute back massage whilst the other group watched television during the same period. The massage group reported feeling better after therapy, and the researchers noted they were 'less fidgety and more co-operative' on the fifth day than they had been at the beginning of the study. However, perhaps more significantly, the massaged group revealed lowered pulse rate and lowered levels of cortisol (a chemical produced under stress) in their saliva – a change that was not noted in any of the television watching group. This study provides data which indicates that massage therapy has positive effects which are clinically measurable. With such conclusive evidence being accumulated by researchers, there seems little doubt that massage therapy does indeed have an important role to play in the future of medicine.

4
COMMON CONDITIONS HELPED BY MASSAGE THERAPY

Massage therapy has beneficial physiological effects on all the major body systems and consequently is commonly used to treat a wide range of diseases, disorders and deformities. Listed below are some of the more common health complaints that massage therapy has been successful in treating.

ANXIETY

Massage therapy is proving to be one of the most successful therapies in the treatment of anxiety. Performed with the appropriate essential oils, it helps relieve accumulated tensions and calms the troubled mind. Indeed, most people who walk into a massage clinic anxious or agitated usually walk out calm and relaxed.

Massage is particularly helpful in those emergencies where someone suffers an anxiety attack because the soothing effect of the hands-on treatment brings with it a unique feeling of care and support for the recipient. It often takes no longer than a few minutes to effectively reduce anxiety in a person. In fact, no one can fail but be comforted by a good massage because the response is instinctive. The slow, firm pressure of controlled strokes gives immediate relief from anxiety in just the same way as a child becomes comforted when being held in a state of agitation.

Massage therapy provides relief from the symptoms of anxiety and gives the patient an opportunity to rest a troubled mind. Often this enables him to reassess the problem later in a calm emotional state which is more conducive to finding solutions to the worries and frustrations which may have caused the anxiety. It is certainly a more preferable method of controlling anxiety than the use of drugs, because some medications can be addictive and cause a plethora of side effects.

Massage therapy helps the patient deal with the physical symptoms of anxiety but massage should not be the only treatment. Psychological problems can often be helped by psychotherapy and counselling. It is always advisable, particularly in cases of chronic anxiety, for the patient to seek help from a counsellor or psychotherapist in order to deal with any unresolved emotional conflicts.

ARTHRITIS

Arthritis is a disorder in which the joints become inflamed. There are two major types of arthritis – osteo-arthritis and rheumatoid arthritis – both require different treatment.

Osteo-arthritis mainly affects the load-bearing joints – the hips, knees and ankles – and usually develops over a long period of time due to wear and tear. Massage therapy consists of helping to cleanse the affected tissues immediately around the joint and strengthening the related muscles. This usually relieves any pain and continued treatment helps keep the condition under control.

Rheumatoid arthritis is a systemic disease affecting all the joints in the body which become inflamed and painful. As the disease progresses, the tissues stiffen and distort in shape.

Whilst massage therapy can help prevent the progress of the disease and alleviate the painful symptoms, comprehensive remedial treatment also requires the consideration of dietary factors and other complementary therapies.

ASTHMA

There may be several factors causing or contributing to the asthma involving diet, stress, as well as environmental and hereditary factors. The bronchial muscles go into spasm in response to irritation of the mucous membranes, and the breathing becomes difficult and laboured. In conventional medicine, it is usually treated by anti-histamine medications which are inhaled or injected. This gives symptomatic relief but does not 'cure' the disease.

Massage therapy helps relieve the symptoms by reducing the general tension of the body and mind. The chest, shoulders and abdomen are the principal areas treated, and therapists often work on the reflex points on the feet and back to help the condition. Acupressure is commonly used and has been known to help clear asthma altogether, but all the possible causes of the condition – e.g. allergens in the home or work-place, an abundance of mucus-forming foods in the diet, or emotional stresses – should be considered in order to find the appropriate permanent remedy.

BACKACHE

A report by the Office of Health Economics has estimated that the treatment of backache costs the National Health Service over £100,000 million every year. One in 20 people consult their GP each year with back problems and it is the single largest cause for absenteeism from work.

Whilst some backaches can be caused by internal troubles such as constipation and kidney infection, over 95 per cent of all backaches are caused by musculo/skeletal disorders. It is therefore little wonder that massage therapy is one of the most effective treatments for backache and back pain. Treatment consists first of relieving the pain and then correcting the cause of the problem, the aim being to reduce the inflammation and then free any restrictions in the vertebrae and surrounding tissues by rebalancing the damaged muscles.

Perhaps more importantly, regular massage therapy will help *prevent* backache. Most people's backs are placed under tremendous strain each day, particularly in an office environment, and massage deals with any adhesions and distortions in the tissues before they can develop into serious problems.

COMMON COLD

Massage can help speed the recovery of a person suffering from colds and influenza by helping to stimulate the body's immune system and by encouraging the elimination of the accumulated toxins. The addition of essential oils (see page 67) in the treatment helps to clear the sinuses and the respiratory tract, and regular massage can also help prevent the onset of colds by ensuring that the toxins are frequently flushed from the tissues and that the immune system is continually stimulated.

CONSTIPATION

Constipation is often caused by tension in the rectal and lower intestinal muscles. Massage to the back and abdomen helps to relax the muscles and so relieve the condition. It also stimulates the peristaltic movement of the intestines, and treatment of the deep tissues can even help clear small blockages in the colon. One woman came to see me who had been suffering from constipation for over 20 years and, after two months of regular treatments combined with a change of diet, she was able to pass regular bowel motions.

CRAMP

Cramp occurs when muscles become over contracted and go into spasm, and is usually caused by an irritated nerve or an imbalance of the minerals in the body. It most frequently affects the calf muscles or the sole of the foot. The pain can be very severe and, at times, excruciating. Typical treatment involves stretching the affected muscle group followed by soothing stroking movements which also help to relax the muscles and thus relieve the pain. Regular massage treatments can also help prevent recurring cramps by ensuring that the muscles are flushed of metabolic wastes.

DEPRESSION

Massage has always been used by people who are feeling low or whose energy levels are down. Massage relaxes, calms and rejuvenates, contributing enormously to a person's sense of well being. In fact, massage has been found to be *so* effective in the treatment of depression, particularly when combined with essential oils, that it is now being incorporated into the treatment of patients suffering from chronic or clinical depression in hospital. The patients are also taught to improve their posture, holding the head up, chest out, and to breathe deeply, because clinical studies have shown that it is almost impossible for a person to 'feel' depressed if he or she is holding his or her body upright, breathing deeply, and smiling. Look around you, and you will see that all 'depressed' people are hunched over the shoulders, looking downwards and breathing very shallowly. However, in severe cases of depression, regular massage treatment should be accompanied by a psychotherapist to get to the root of the problem and so speed a full recovery.

FROZEN SHOULDER (CAPSULITIS)

Frozen shoulders is thought to be caused by lesions in the tissues around the joint capsule which create inflammation in the area. It makes most movement of the arm or shoulder very painful and, in some cases, the shoulder becomes almost totally immobilised (hence the term 'frozen'). Moving the arm upwards or behind your back is particularly difficult, and consequently this means that most household chores and everyday domestic activities including such things as brushing your hair or picking up the telephone can become a major problem, being almost impossible to do using the affected arm.

A frozen shoulder usually lasts for about 18 months and then often disappears spontaneously, leaving as quickly as it came. No one is really sure how and why this happens. However, during that period, massage therapy can help ease the pain and keep the shoulder area as flexible as possible. It also encourages a faster recovery by improving blood flow to the area and breaking down any adhesions formed in the soft tissues.

HEADACHES

Headaches may have a variety of causes ranging from food intolerances, eye strain, digestive disturbances, muscular tension or a displaced vertebra in the neck. However, most headaches occur from subluxations (partial dislocation) in the vertebrae of the neck, or tension in the neck and shoulder muscles, which create a build-up of pressure in the head.

It is for this reason that massage therapy is very effective in treating headaches. Treatment to the upper back, neck and shoulders not only affords fast relief from headaches and migraine but regular massage treatments also help prevent the onset of headaches by keeping the neck and shoulder muscles balanced and relaxed.

HIGH BLOOD PRESSURE

High blood pressure can be caused by several factors, the two major causes being narrowed arteries and emotional stress. The narrowing of the arteries is caused by cholesterol and mineral deposits building up on the arterial walls which can significantly increase blood pressure. In this instance, changes in the diet are essential to reduce the intake of cholesterol into the body. Moreover, certain foods – including garlic, oats and lecithin – have been found, in clinical studies, to reduce cholesterol levels in the blood stream significantly.

However, many cases of high blood pressure are brought about by emotional stress, which causes the muscles to contract and constrict the arteries. A simple back massage or neck and shoulder treatment can, within a few minutes, release the tightness in the tissues and has a reflex effect on the nervous system. In these cases massage has a profound and immediate effect on the blood pressure.

Regular massage is very effective in controlling high blood pressure caused through tension and, in the first instance, should be considered as an alternative to conventional drug therapy. Many medications prescribed to control high blood pressure can have unpleasant side effects, such as dizziness, muscle cramps, fatigue and impaired kidney function and often need to be continued fo the rest of the patient's life.

However, if blood pressure is already being controlled through medication, you should consult your GP before commencing any alternative therapies.

INSOMNIA

Massage is an excellent remedy for insomnia because it has the ability to send a person into a deep sleep within a short space of time. It is, of course, one of the safest remedies, far preferable to sleeping pills many of which can be habit-forming as well as having unpleasant side effects. Many patients have come to me because of a bad backache or neck pain who later commented that the treatments had not only relieved their pains, but had also enabled them to sleep much better.

An evening massage given just before retiring to bed enables most people who suffer from insomnia to sleep soundly, and it even seems to help the person giving the massage too. Clare Maxwell-Hudson wrote of an 11-year-old girl who was brought to her suffering from insomnia. 'I taught the mother how to massage her daughter. This not only helped the girl to sleep, but also calmed the mother. That is the wonderful thing about massage ... it works both ways and can be of equal benefit to the giver and the receiver.'

In cases of insomnia Dr William Murrel MD, FRCP advises: 'General massage at bed-time undoubtedly promotes sleep. The result is not only certain but prompt, the patient usually enjoying a good night's rest after the first seance. It has the advantage over all narcotics that there are no disagreeable side effects.'

MUSCLE STRAIN

In my experience no other therapy or medicine can better massage in the treatment of muscular strain. It will remedy the injured tissue and ensure that there are no residual problems with the muscle. If a muscle strain is not treated, it can lead to a chronic arthritic disorder because the muscle fibres become imbalanced and slowly pull the joint out of its correct position.

For example, a muscle strain in the lower back can, if neglected, result in lumbar vertebrae becoming displaced and this, in turn, puts pressure on the inter-vertebral discs and the related nerve roots. The person will then need continuous treatment to ease the pressure on the nerve and so control the pain.

OEDEMA

Oedema (fluid retention) can occur following an injury or from poor lymphatic circulation. Massage is probably the most effective means of helping to drain away accumulated lymph and body fluids. The most typical form of oedema occurs to the ankles, and massage to the legs, commencing at the top of the thigh, is extremely effective in stimulating the flow of lymph and thus reducing the swelling.

One patient, who had sprained his ankle in a football match, ended up with a swelling measuring over 14 inches in circumference, nearly double its normal size. With 10 days of continuous treatment accompanied by hydrotherapy footbaths the swelling was reduced and the ankle returned to its original size.

RECOVERY FROM AN ILLNESS

We have all experienced how, during a bout of flu, our bodies ache and feel weak. Toxins begin to accumulate in the tissues of the body and slowly these need to be eliminated. Massage cleanses the tissues of these metabolic wastes and in so doing aids recovery. I conducted a small study in my clinic with some of my patients. I asked them to test their urine in the morning and evening on the day before having massage treatment, then again on the following day before and after the treatment. The nitrogenous wastes, inorganic salts and ketones (fat waste products) in the urine were higher in the afternoon than in the morning but were higher still after the massage, demonstrating the cleansing effect of massage therapy.

RHEUMATISM

The term rheumatism means 'pain in the soft tissues'. This is often substantially alleviated by massage therapy which releases any restrictions in the tissues and cleanses the tissues of lactic acid and other metabolic wastes. I cannot recall one patient suffering from rheumatism who did not greatly benefit from massage therapy. However, massage only alleviates the symptoms and, as in all health problems, it is important to look to the cause of the condition whether dietetic or physical, and then take appropriate remedial action.

SCIATICA

True sciatica is a very painful condition indeed, characterised by sharp, shooting pains down one or both legs. It is often so painful that the person becomes temporarily bedridden, being unable to walk or even to stand. It is caused by pressure on the sciatic nerve running through the buttock and down the legs.

Bed rest is essential in all cases of sciatica and the inflammation should be allowed to subside before any form of treatment is started. Massage initially relaxes the muscles and eases the pressure on the nerve to alleviate the pain and the massage therapist will then continue by rebalancing the tissues and thus prevent recurrence.

STRESS

See Chapter 12.

TENDINITIS

Tendinitis means inflammation of a tendon. The tendons attach muscle to the bone and they may become inflamed if the major muscle groups are strained or the joint is displaced by a traumatic injury.

Many physiotherapists use ultrasound wave therapy on the damaged tendon but massage therapy focuses primarily on the muscles that attach to the injured tendon rather than concentrating on the tendon itself and there are sound reasons for this approach to the treatment. If any tendon is inflamed, then it is more than likely that the muscle to which the tendon is attached will also be affected and, as it is the muscles that pull the tendon, the muscles need to be relaxed and any adhesions within the muscle tissues removed before effective treatment can be given to the tendon itself.

One young girl who came to see me about a particularly severe case of tendinitis in the achilles tendons of both legs had been given ultrasound treatment by her physiotherapist for six months. But the treatment had been limited to the ultrasound on the tendons with no treatment at all to the calf or leg muscles.

I asked her what she had been doing immediately prior to the onset of the pain in her legs and she said that she had been on a long hike. This confirmed that there had been muscular strain. Very often when a muscle is strained, the point at which

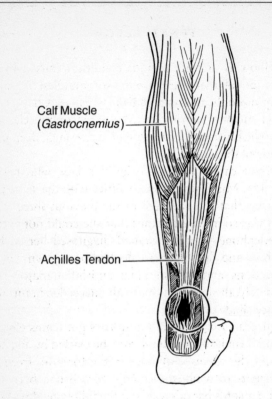

Calf Muscle
(*Gastrocnemius*)

Achilles Tendon

Achilles Tendinitis

we feel pain is the point where the muscle attaches to the tendon. If, for example, you were to glue a piece of rope to the wall and then pull it, the point at which it is most likely to break is where it is stuck to the wall. In human anatomy, that is the tendon attachment.

Examination of her lower limbs confirmed to me that the problem in her tendons was related to her calf muscles which were both stiff and contained numerous adhesions. I immediately massaged her legs, and simply by breaking up the adhesions and cleansing the tissues, she was free of the pain within three sessions.

TENNIS ELBOW

Tennis elbow is another painful condition caused by acute inflammation of the forearm extensor muscles. A common complaint not only afficting tennis players (see Chapter 11), it can affect anyone who strains the extensor muscles in the forearm. The muscles become inflamed causing a deep pain on the outside of the elbow.

The worst case I ever saw was of a lady who had been baking cakes. Mrs B arrived at my office with the same pain in her forearms that she had had for the previous three months. The pain was so intense at times that she could not even pick up the telephone. Her doctor had diagnosed her as having tennis elbow and the treatment she had been given was cortisone injections and non-steroidal anti-inflammatory drugs. Unfortunately, the injections had only succeeded in turning her arms a nice shade of purple.

How had a woman in her mid-forties got tennis elbow you might ask? Tennis elbow can, in fact, be caused by any activity that strains the extensor muscles in the forearm, from lifting heavy weights to window cleaning. Mrs B had been baking cakes for her son's bar mitzvah and the following day she felt a terrible ache in her arms.

Anti-inflammatory injections may help initially to reduce inflammation but they do not get to the root of the problem and therefore cannot help the muscle to heal. In fact, with the help of pain killers Mrs B only succeeded in aggravating her condition. Pain is the body's way of telling us to stop and let the muscle rest; killing the pain enables a person to continue to use the damaged muscle and, as a result, the underlying problem will then worsen.

If a condition is seen by a massage therapist shortly after the injury, the treatment will work faster than if it is left for weeks or months. This is because any excessive lymph hardens and causes the muscle fibres to stick together forming adhesions.

Once adhesions are formed it can be a long and often painful process to get rid of them.

Working first with reflexes in the feet to help reduce the inflammation, I then massaged Mrs B's neck and upper arms to help clear away accumulated lymph and cleanse the tissues before doing the same with the wrist. It was only then that we were finally able to slowly treat the injured forearms and, although it took a few months, the condition was eventually cleared.

Massage treatment of tennis elbow

The aim of massage therapy in the case of tennis elbow is to first reduce the inflammation and then cleanse and rebalance the forearm muscles. The inflammation is treated with ice and the massage therapist treats the neck and upper arm muscles. Slowly, the massage therapist works down to the forearm muscles which are often most tender near the tendon attachment to the elbow.

All massage treatment involves the neck, upper back and upper arm, in addition to the forearm itself, in order to ensure that there is no nerve restriction in the neck or arm which may have caused or contributed to the onset of the condition.

In all cases of tennis elbow it is important to seek help as soon as possible because continuous irritation can result in calcification forming around the tendons which could require surgery to rectify. The sooner treatment is commenced, the sooner the problem will be rectified, and any problem neglected for too long can take months or even years to remedy.

TINNITUS

Tinnitus is the continuous ringing in the ears for which there is no known cure. However, manipulation of the ears and the surrounding muscles often provides effective relief by alleviating any physical pressures, and acupressure techniques have been known to eliminate the condition altogether.

TORTICOLLIS

Torticollis (wry neck) occurs when the muscles in one side of the neck go into spasm forcing the neck to tilt sideways. This can be a very painful condition and in severe cases may require corrective surgery. Massage is often used to help treat this condition by relaxing the spasmed tissues and later strengthening and balancing the neck and shoulder muscles. Heat treatment is used to help relax the tissues and a neck collar is often required to keep the vertebrae in the neck supported in their correct position and to give temporary relief to the strained muscles.

VARICOSE VEINS

Massage can be of great benefit to a person suffering with varicose veins. Massage stimulates the venous blood flow and thereby reduces the pressure on the veins caused by the incompetent valves inside the veins. However, it is contra-indicated to massage directly over varicose veins because it may irritate them or cause them to worsen. Light massage should be commenced above the bulging vein and then below.

Regular massage is an excellent preventive measure which can help prevent the formation of varicose veins and, where they already exist, massage will help prevent the condition from worsening.

5

THE PHYSIOLOGY OF MASSAGE THERAPY AND HOW IT AFFECTS THE BODY SYSTEMS

Massage has beneficial physiological effects on all of the major systems in the body, some of which have been shown to be measurable in clinical studies. In order to appreciate the value of massage therapy in helping to treat a health problem, it is important to understand just what these benefits on the body systems are, and how they are produced.

MASSAGE AND MUSCLES

Muscles are perhaps the tissues in the body most talked about and least understood. There are over 500 different muscles throughout the body and together they do much more than merely help us run around a tennis court or play a round of golf. Virtually every bodily function depends upon muscular action in one way or another. Walking, talking, smiling, breathing, seeing and even digesting food could not be done without muscles.

Muscles are known as 'contractile' tissue because they function by contracting and thereby create movement. They are attached to the bones via the tendons which are stronger and more fibrous tissue. Most muscles work in pairs so that when one muscle is flexed the corresponding (antagonistic) muscle is stretched. This you can easily experience by fully flexing the bicep muscle in the upper arm and noticing how the tricep muscle on the other side of the arm is being stretched. The two opposing muscle groups therefore contract and pull in opposite directions but in so doing create a perfect balance. It is only when that natural balance becomes disturbed through one muscle becoming too flaccid and weak or another becoming too tense or in spasm that we begin to experience muscle-related disorders such as visceroptosis (a condition in which the abdominal organs drop downward caused by weak abdominal muscles), torticolis (wry neck), or tennis elbow.

Although massage has been used as a therapeutic technique by physical therapists for a long time, substantiation of its effects on muscle relaxation and a scientific basis for this reputed effect had been lacking. But recent research has

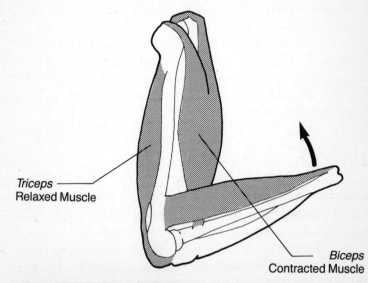

Triceps
Relaxed Muscle

Biceps
Contracted Muscle

BALANCING MUSCLE GROUPS

suggested that petrissage (kneading massage) of muscles inhibits the activity of the muscle's spinal motor neurons, causing the muscles to relax. Other techniques such as tendon pressure or tapping on muscles have also been found to reduce motor-neuron excitability, again causing a decrease in muscle tension.

To better understand the effects of massage on the neuro-muscular system, a study was conducted using 16 subjects (eight male and eight female) who were massaged on four sites on their legs. As in most studies of this type, changes in what is called the 'H-reflex amplitude' – an indirect measure of motor-neuron excitability – were monitored by studying the electrical signals in muscles. The results were the same on all of the subjects and, as with other techniques for stretching muscles, petrissage brought about decreased motor-neuron activity in the massaged muscle. Inhibition of the muscle in the calf was not observed when massage was given in the thigh or on two areas on the other leg. The study indicates clearly that massage reduces muscle reflex activity specifically in the muscle being massaged.

There are two main types of muscle in the human body – voluntary muscles (e.g. the muscles in your leg which contract as and when you consciously tell them to) and involuntary muscles (e.g. the intestinal wall), which are co-ordinated by the brain without your conscious direction.

VOLUNTARY MUSCLES

Massage is commonly used to help treat many muscular dis-orders affecting the voluntary muscles which range from muscular strain to rheumatism. This is because massage increases blood flow, helps cleanse the tissues of accumulated metabolic wastes, and breaks down any muscular adhesions (muscle fibres stuck together with hardened lymph fluid). In doing so, massage also helps to tone muscles and prevent muscle wasting.

Muscles can deteriorate very quickly. Bind up your left arm for a few days and then compare it with the right arm. You will see how, even in such a short time, the muscles on the left arm have already begun to waste. The US Airforce recently carried out an interesting study; they took a group of their fittest men and laid them up in bed for two weeks. They then put them back into the normal routine to see how long it would take for these men to get back to their original level of fitness. It took three months. Imagine, if it takes three months to recover from just two weeks of a sedentary lifestyle, what would a year or years of doing little or no exercise do to a person's general fitness and muscular strength? It is not difficult to appreciate how important exercise is to maintain strong and healthy muscle tissue.

Whilst massage is no substitute for exercise, it can improve the tone of the tissues and help prevent muscle wasting where exercise is not possible. If a patient suffers from paralysis or any other chronic debilitating illness, or if he or she is simply laid up in bed with a bad back, massage is an excellent form of remedial treatment helping prevent further decline in the patient's muscle tissues and, in many cases, promoting strength.

INVOLUNTARY MUSCLES

Massage is also being frequently used to treat the involuntary muscles due to the reflex effect it has on those muscles through the nervous system. A speeding heart beat, twitching eyelids, or sluggish intestines can all be improved with massage therapy.

INJURIES

We have all suffered some form of muscular injury in our lives. It is difficult to go through life without taking a few knocks and bumps along the way. Whether we are kicked in the leg during a football game or are hit in the ankle by a supermarket trolley, the muscles are injured and as a result are weakened. In many cases, the body's healing mechanisms act quickly and there is no lasting problem. But, if a person has poor circulation, the healing process is often hindered and he or she ends up with a chronic problem.

A groin strain can persist for years, as can a bad back. The reason for this is that after any injury, a fluid called 'lymph' travels to the injured tissues to bathe and nourish them, and remove any waste products as they heal. The lymph is then circulated through lymphatic vessels, much like veins, to lymph nodes where any harmful bacteria are eliminated.

If the lymph travels too slowly, it becomes sticky, attaching itself to the surrounding tissues and then hardens. Injured muscle fibres can end up stuck together in knots by the hardened lymph creating 'adhesions' which is when we can feel the muscle 'knotted up' and as a result the muscle group is weakened.

Muscles work on an 'all or nothing' principle – a muscle fibre either contracts fully or not at all. So, if a muscle has, say, 100 fibres it only uses those fibres it needs. At any one time there may be less than 50 actually working unless we are exerting ourselves, in which case there may be 90 or even 100 contracted. Therefore a muscle will often cope long after an injury and will only create pain when the damaged fibres are required to work. This is why we sometimes get a pain in the same area every now and again. The 'now and again' being those times when we need to use the damaged muscle fibres.

Massage actually helps the body to recover from injuries because the movement helps to cleanse the tissues and aids blood and lymph circulation, and in doing so, it helps prevent lymph congestion and the formation of muscular adhesions and scar tissue.

JOINTS

Massage is also very effective in helping all sorts of problems relating to joints. After all, the muscles and soft tissues hold a joint in its correct position. If muscles are damaged, they must, sooner or later, affect the joint to which they are attached. The muscles can either pull the joint out of position or compress the bones together, creating pressure inside the joint. Re-balancing the muscles will therefore help the joint to return to its correct, stress-free position.

But massage has a further impact on the condition of the joints through the nervous system. There is a law in physiology called Hilton's Law which states that the nerve that enervates a muscle also affects the joint to which the muscle is attached. It has therefore been established that any treatment of the muscle will also affect the joint itself because the nerve supplying the joint is stimulated. It is for this reason that we witness such remarkable results in massage therapy in helping treat many joint disorders including rheumatoid and osteo-arthritis.

POOR POSTURE

The way we stand, the way we sit, the way we walk are all what is commonly referred to as posture. If we stand hunched over looking at the floor instead of straight ahead, we strain the upper back muscles as well as the neck and shoulders, the abdominal muscles sag, the diaphragm becomes weak and we breathe less deeply. Ailments directly affected by the strains of poor posture include digestive disorders, breathing difficulties, migraines and tension headaches as well as backache. Poor posture is difficult to correct unless some form of remedial therapy is sought. There are various therapies that do help including yoga and the Alexander Technique, and massage can also help this process by strengthening the loose tissues and relaxing any tight muscles.

THE CARDIO-VASCULAR SYSTEM

The cardio-vascular system comprises the heart, the blood and the blood vessels (arteries and veins) through which the blood is transported. The blood nourishes the rest of the body by distributing nutrients and oxygen, and then cleanses the tissues by removing the waste products produced by the body cells.

The blood is pumped by the heart through the arteries and into the smaller vessels called 'capillaries' which have permeable walls enabling the nutrients and oxygen in the blood to pass through to the cells of the organs and body tissues. Carbon dioxide and other waste products are collected in the capillaries, passed into the veins, and then transported back to the heart.

Although blood is pumped through the arteries by the heart, the blood's journey back to the heart through the veins requires muscle contraction to push it upwards against the force of gravity. The veins are endowed with valves which prevent the downward flow of blood. It is when these valves lose their strength that the blood is allowed to flow downward and consequently the vein bulges and becomes varicosed.

Massage improves the blood circulation in several ways without putting any additional strain on the heart. The direct pressure during massage therapy on the blood vessels helps to push the blood through the veins and also stimulates the nerves which control the blood vessels. It also has the added benefit of relaxing any tense muscles or tight connective tissue which may have been constricting the blood vessels, enabling the blood to flow more freely. Soothing massage also reduces emotional tension, inducing relaxation, and thereby calms stress-related cardio-vascular conditions including tachycardia (spasmodic and abnormally rapid heart beats), arrythmia (disturbance of the heart's rhythm), and high blood pressure.

In the last century, Sir Lauder Brunton, a Victorian cardiologist, said: 'In cases of cardiac disease, massage allows other treatments to be carried out more easily'. In recent years massage has been shown to be so helpful in the treatment of patients suffering from cardiovascular disorders that it is being commonly prescribed to help treat patients suffering from heart-related and circulatory diseases.

THE DIGESTIVE SYSTEM

The digestive system consists of the mouth, gullet, stomach and intestines, as well as the digestive organs – the liver, gall bladder and pancreas. All of these organs are affected by the conditions of the muscles and other tissue surrounding them.

If you were to sit in an operating theatre and watch a surgeon perform an abdominal operation, one of the first things you would notice is how all of the internal organs are moving to a certain rhythm created by the abdominal muscles. If the abdominal muscles are too weak, the organs lose their natural rhythm and become sluggish, and if the muscles are too tense the organs and intestines become constricted leading to conditions such as colic, constipation, irritable bowel syndrome and the like.

Massage is, therefore, an excellent therapy which will help most digestive disorders (except inflammatory conditions such as gastritis or colitis) because it can help relax or strengthen abdominal muscles. It has also been recorded that manipulating the tissues of the abdomen can promote secretion by the digestive glands and so aid digestion. Increased blood flow to the abdomen will improve the assimilation of nutrients into the blood stream. Massage over the large intestine stimulates the peristalsic action of the intestines – the wave-like contractions of the intestinal walls – which moves food through the gut and assists the excretion of faeces from the bowels. As such, massage can be invaluable in relieving constipation.

THE LYMPHATIC SYSTEM

The lymphatic system is an extension of the blood circulation and is often referred to as the waste disposal system of the body. The lymph vessels, like veins, transport the lymph fluid in one direction only, in this case towards the lymph glands rather than the heart.

It works in this way: blood plasma seeps through the walls of the capillaries to nourish and bathe tissues and then drains into lymph vessels taking with it waste products from the cells. This 'lymph' is carried through the lymph vessels towards the lymphatic glands – situated in the armpits, groin, neck, base of the lungs and around the intestines – where it is filtered and any bacteria is destroyed. If, for instance, you are cut or injured, germs may enter the wound but the body responds by activating its immune system. The germs will be trapped in the lymph vessel, transported to the lymph nodes where they are destroyed.

If the lymphatic system were to stop working you would be dead within a day. In the same way that massage stimulates the venous blood flow, it also encourages the flow of lymph through the body and, in doing so, helps eliminate body wastes, reduce any oedema (fluid retention) and swelling.

If you are injured, the massage therapist works on the area above the injury first to ensure that the lymph will be able to flow and then on the site of the swelling itself. Massage significantly improves the flow of lymph through the body and thereby speeds up the recovery of an injury. When coupled with light, daily exercise, regular massage treatment has also substantially reduced and even eliminated the puffy and swollen ankles associated with water retention from which so many women suffer.

THE SKIN

The skin is the largest organ in the body and is often terribly abused, choked with make-up and suffocated by synthetic clothing materials, so it is no surprise that so many people have skin complaints. The skin is not simply a protective coating, preventing germs from entering the body, it helps to regulate the body temperature and it also eliminates toxins from the body through perspiration.

Massage helps to nourish and recondition the skin, and it also stimulates elimination through the skin by bringing a greater concentration of blood to the outer skin layers. It is also often of great benefit to stress-related skin disorders such as psoriasis and eczema. However, you should not have massage therapy if you are suffering from any skin condition without first consulting your medical doctor.

RESPIRATORY SYSTEM

Massage has been considered for many years to be an important form of treatment for many respiratory disorders. Patients hospitalised with conditions such as bronchopneumonia and bronchiectasis, where the lungs and bronchials secrete excess mucous or pus, receive percussion massage to help eliminate the congestion. Many essential oils including cedarwood, camphor, mint and cinamon are now commonly used to further help clear the nasal and bronchial passageways.

Massage is also used to help treat stress-related respiratory diseases including asthma. Many respiratory disorders are caused or augmented by tightness of the muscles and a constricted chest. In asthma, for instance, the bronchial tubes go into spasm making it difficult for the sufferer to exhale. When we are stressed, our chest muscles are tensed and we tend to breathe very shallowly. If the abdominal muscles are constantly tense, the diaphragm is unable to fully expand or relax and often over a long period of time, the breathing suffers.

Massage helps by reducing general tension and also specific muscular tensions. Acupressure techniques can also affect the lungs themselves through the same points as those used in acupuncture. By massaging the outside of the body, we can actually create a beneficial response inside the body. Furthermore, when massage is combined with aromatherapy essential oils, it can also help clear and relax the respiratory tract.

NERVOUS SYSTEM

The nervous system is perhaps the most complex and mysterious system in the body, controlling all of the other body systems. It is in essence an extremely intricate system of channels through which messages between the brain and the rest of the body are sent and received. It is analogous to a complex electrical circuit that serves and controls all organs and tissues in the body.

The nervous system begins with the brain and extends down the spinal cord in the back from where it branches out to the rest of the body. Each branch (otherwise known as nerve roots) stemming from the spinal cord travels to a different part of the body. In order for the body's tissues to remain healthy they must receive adequate blood supply and also sufficient nerve supply. If the vertebrae in the spine become displaced, they can press on the nerve root and restrict the nerve supply. As a result the area of the body that should be receiving nerve supply from that nerve root is deprived and weakens.

Disease is often a result. The chart below shows how the numerous nerve roots in the spinal column affect the rest of the body, and how, if restricted over any length of time, they can actually cause diseases affecting the lungs, the stomach and the heart, besides weakening other muscles.

This is the underlying principle of chiropractic and osteopathic treatments which manipulate the joints throughout the body and particularly in the spine in order to free any restrictions in the nerve fibres and blood vessels. Massage therapy also helps to free restricted nerve roots and, more importantly, helps to keep them unrestricted.

A few years ago I was consulted by a young optician who had originally come to see me about a sprained ankle. After a few treatments the ankle was put to rights, but during his final treatment I noticed that the left side of his face seemed a little stiff. At the end of the appointment he mentioned that several years ago he had suffered from Bell's palsy (facial paralysis), a nervous disorder which had caused one side of his face to stay paralysed for several months before it began to recover. However, he was now beginning to experience the same symptoms as he had had all those years ago and, quite naturally, he was very worried. Apart from having to talk to people in his optometry practice, he was getting married that same year.

I examined his neck and shoulders and found his muscles were extremely tense especially on the left side which could be affecting the blood flow and restricting the nerve pathways. I suggested that he have two massage treatments to try and loosen the tissues and see if this affected his facial condition. He agreed and, two days after the first treatment, he telephoned my office to say that not only did his neck feel freer than it had done for years, but that the symptoms affecting his

Vertebrae	Area Controlled by Nerves*	Possible Effects of a Malfunction
1C	Blood supply to the head, pituitary gland, scalp, bones of the face, brain, inner and middle ear, sympathetic nervous system.	☐ headaches, ☐ nervousness, ☐ insomnia, ☐ head colds, ☐ high blood pressure, ☐ migraine headaches, ☐ chronic tiredness, ☐ dizziness.
2C	Eyes, optic nerves, auditory nerves, sinuses, mastoid bones, tongue, forehead.	☐ sinus trouble, ☐ allergies, ☐ pain around the eyes, ☐ earache, ☐ fainting spells, ☐ deafness.
3C	Cheeks, outer ear, face bones, teeth, tri-facial nerve.	☐ neuralgia, ☐ neuritis.
4C	Nose, lips, mouth, eustachian tube.	☐ runny nose, ☐ hearing loss.
5C	Vocal cords, neck glands, pharynx.	☐ laryngitis, ☐ hoarseness, ☐ throat conditions such as sore throat.
6C	Neck muscles, shoulders, tonsils.	☐ stiff neck, ☐ pain in upper arm, ☐ tonsillitis, ☐ chronic cough.
7C	Thyroid gland, bursae in the shoulders, elbows.	☐ bursitis, ☐ colds, ☐ thyroid conditions.
1T	Arms from the elbows down, including hands, wrists, and fingers; oesophagus and trachea.	☐ cough, ☐ difficult breathing or shortness of breath, ☐ pain in lower arms and hands.
2T	Heart, including its valves and coverings; coronary arteries.	☐ functional heart conditions and certain chest conditions.
3T	Lungs, bronchial tubes, pleura, chest, breast.	☐ bronchitis, ☐ pleurisy, ☐ pneumonia, ☐ congestion, ☐ influenza.
4T	Gall bladder, common duct.	☐ gall bladder conditions.
5T	Liver, solar plexus, circulation (general).	☐ liver conditions, ☐ blood pressure problems, ☐ poor circulation.
6T	Stomach.	☐ stomach troubles or nervous stomach, ☐ indigestion, ☐ heartburn, ☐ dyspepsia.

NECK REGION (1C–7C)

MID-BACK

ATLAS
AXIS

CERVICAL
SPINE

1st
THORACIC

Vertebra	Body part	Region	Conditions / Symptoms
7T	Pancreas, duodenum.		☐ ulcers, ☐ gastritis.
8T	Spleen.		☐ lowered resistance.
9T	Adrenal and supra-renal glands.		☐ allergies, ☐ hives.
10T	Kidneys.		☐ kidney troubles, ☐ chronic tiredness, ☐ nephritis, ☐ pyelitis.
11T	Kidneys, ureters.		☐ skin conditions such as acne, ☐ pimples, ☐ eczema, ☐ or boils.
12T	Small intestines, lymph circulation.		☐ rheumatism, ☐ gas pains.
1L	Large intestines, inguinal rings.	LOW BACK	☐ constipation, ☐ colitis, ☐ diarrhoea.
2L	Appendix, abdomen, upper leg.	LOW BACK	☐ cramps, ☐ difficult breathing, ☐ minor varicose veins.
3L	Sex organs, uterus, bladder, knees.	LOW BACK	☐ bladder troubles, ☐ menstrual troubles such as painful or irregular periods, ☐ change of life symptoms, ☐ many knee pains.
4L	Prostate gland, muscles of the lower back, sciatic nerve.	LOW BACK	☐ sciatica, ☐ lumbago, ☐ difficult, painful, or too frequent urination, ☐ backaches.
5L	Lower legs, ankles, feet.	LOW BACK	☐ poor circulation in the legs, ☐ swollen ankles, weak ankles and arches, ☐ cold feet, ☐ weakness in the legs, ☐ leg cramps.
SACRUM	Hip bones, buttocks.	PELVIS	☐ sacro-iliac conditions, ☐ spinal curvatures.
COCCYX	Rectum, anus.		☐ pain at end of spine on sitting.

THORACIC SPINE
1st LUMBAR
LUMBAR SPINE
SACRUM
COCCYX

*Directly or indirectly controlled

face had significantly improved also. During the second treatment we were able to work on the deeper muscles and, before the week was up, all signs of the facial paralysis had gone.

All spinal joints (vertebrae and intervertebral discs) are held in place only by the soft tissues around them – the muscles, tendons and ligaments. Therefore if a joint has become displaced without traumatic injury – i.e. without falling over or being hit by a shopping trolley – then it must have become displaced through an imbalance in the muscles. It is much like a tent pole being held in place by two pieces of rope. If one rope is tighter than the other, the pole will tilt out of position. You can push the pole back in place, but if one rope still remains tighter than the other one, it will pull the pole straight out of position again.

Certainly, adjustment of bones is necessary when the joints are chronically displaced or under acute trauma; but the soft tissues will still require treatment because they will also have been distorted. The bones are continuously moving, all day, every day, pulled by the muscles and tendons. It is for this reason that I believe massage therapy, in conjunction with chiropractice or osteopathy, to be vastly superior to spinal manipulations alone. An adjustment alone might put the joint back into correct alignment, but as soon as you get off the treatment couch your spine will move, and if the tissues around them are not balanced, the vertebrae will be pulled out of place again very quickly. Massage strengthens and rebalances the muscles, and if they are balanced the joint has nowhere else to go but back into its correct position.

Apart from being able to influence the nerve roots in the spine, massage therapy also affects the sensory and motor nerves in the muscles themselves by regulating the nerve reflex activity in the muscle. Coupled with this, massage relaxes the whole central nervous system, and it is for this reason that the nervous system responds so well to the treatment. Massage therapy is used in many nervous disorders, from the chronic degenerative multiple sclerosis and motor neurone disease to numbness, burning sensations and even pins and needles.

6

VISITING A MASSAGE THERAPIST

The good massage therapist can create a relationship which shows the patient how to get well.

Dr Peter Nixon, Consultant Cardiologist,
Charing Cross Hospital, London.

FINDING A PRACTITIONER

Finding a reputable and qualified massage therapist is not always as easy as it might sound. To begin with, phonebook listings do not always separate the trained practitioners from the untrained. So most people find their therapists by word-of-mouth. Contact friends, your doctor, or another health therapist you trust, and ask if they can recommend a practitioner to you. If none of the people you know can offer any leads, my advice is to call or write to one of the registered body of massage therapists (see appendix) and they should be able to provide you with a list of registered massage therapists in your area. Whatever you do, be very careful if you decide to answer adverts in local newspapers as it is still common, and unfortunately not illegal, for prostitutes to offer their services under the guise of massage.

In the UK, there are at present no government regulatory bodies governing the training and ethics of the practice of massage therapists, although EC directives are expected to be implemented in due course. There are numerous massage schools (see appendix) offering varying degrees of training and different qualifications. The oldest teaching institute in the UK is the Northern Institute of Massage (N.I.M) which has trained literally thousands of professional massage therapists for over seventy years. They maintain a register of qualified practitioners and practising massage therapists who have graduated from the N.I.M are governed by the code of conduct of the London & Counties Society of Physiologists – a body established in 1919 to promote massage therapy.

In some other parts of the world massage therapy is governed by statute ensuring that all massage therapists have reached a minimum standard of practice and, just as important, that therapists comply with a professional code of ethics and practice. In Canada, for instance, the Ontario Massage Therapists Association maintains a register and enforces a code of practice for its members, and only their members are allowed by law to promote themselves as 'massage therapists'. This is in stark contrast to the position in the UK where anybody can promote themselves as anything except to call themselves a 'doctor'.

When you do manage to find a massage therapist it is prudent to telephone the practitioner and ask them about their practice, qualifications, and of course, their charges before making an appointment.

THE FIRST APPOINTMENT

Visting a massage therapist is much the same as visiting any other physical therapist whether it be a chiropractor, osteopath or physiotherapist. The clinic will have a treatment couch, heat lamps and fresh towels.

The first appointment will usually involve a detailed consultation to ensure that massage therapy can help your condition and that it is not contra-indicated for any reason.

The therapist will begin by taking a full case history asking questions about:

- Your symptoms – e.g. how long you have had them, when they occur, etc.
- Any other treatment you may be having for the symptoms.
- Any previous treatment you may have had for the symptoms.
- Any medications you may have taken or are presently taking.
- Any surgery you may have had.
- Any known diseases and disorders you may have.
- Whether you are under the care or supervision of your doctor or hospital for any other medical condition.
- Any matters which may make massage therapy contraindicated e.g. pregnancy, infectious skin diseases, etc. (see Chapter 7).
- Your general lifestyle.
- Your family history.

It is a good idea to take written notes of these matters with you as this will save time and ensure that you can provide the therapist with the answers at the first appointment.

The therapist will then conduct a physical examination to determine the state of the muscles and the range of movement of the joints, as well as the general condition of your body. This will involve asking you to do certain movements and then the therapist will palpate (examine by feel) the muscles.

The examination isolates the site of any injuries and determines the most appropriate mode of treatment. As explained in earlier chapters, the site of pain is not always the area requiring treatment. The pain may be referred from another part of the body. For instance, a numbness or burning sensation in the leg is often caused by a restriction of a nerve root in the lower back. Similarly, a pain in the lower back may be caused by a distorted knee or ankle joint.

The consultation and physical examination will provide the massage therapist with a complete picture and he or she will then be able to explain the proposed course of treatment and answer the most common and important questions relating to your symptoms.

- What is causing the problem?
- How long will it take to get better?
- What has to be done in order to get better?
- How can I prevent it happening again?

THE TREATMENT

Once you are satisfied with the therapist's proposed course of treatment the real work begins. A typical treatment usually lasts between 20 minutes and an hour depending upon the nature of the problem. The therapist will tell you what clothes need to be removed and you should be given complete privacy to undress as necessary and cover yourself in a fresh towel or body gown ready for the massage.

Throughout the treatment the massage therapist should ensure that all of your body is covered with a fresh towel except for the area being worked upon. No part of the body is exposed at any time unless it is a necessary part of the treatment. This is not purely to protect the patient's modesty. It is done to ensure that you are relaxed and comfortable throughout the treatment and that all of your body is kept warm.

Is there any pain?

Although there may be times during the treatment when you will experience a little pain, it is pain that most people tend to enjoy because they can feel a sense of release as tense muscle fibres relax and the tissues are cleansed. A therapeutic massage should be a thoroughly relaxing and very enjoyable experience.

PREVENTIVE MEDICINE

Massage therapy is much more than a remedial treatment helping to rid the body of aches and pains, it is also an excellent form of preventive medicine. Most people seem to enjoy a massage and benefit from it far beyond relief of their symptoms. As a result, they usually continue with regular treatments as a preventive measure to keep the effects of stress at bay and maintain a healthy body rather than trying at intervals to repair a sick or injured one.

MEDICAL INSURANCE COVER

Some medical insurance policies will pay for part or all of the cost of your massage therapy, and so it is worth contacting your insurance company to find out if your treatment is covered, and if so, to what extent before commencing treatments. In the UK, most insurers who will pay for massage therapy in their policies do so only if it is recommended by a consultant. However, in Canada and Australia, for instance, massage therapy is covered by many medical insurance policies and insurers allow policy holders to have a certain number of hours treatment without a doctor's certificate.

7

WHEN NOT TO MASSAGE – THE CONTRA-INDICATIONS

Massage is one of the safest therapies available. However, there are times when it is not appropriate to massage and when, in fact, it may be positively harmful and even dangerous. In such circumstances massage is contra-indicated and it is important before giving or receiving a massage treatment to ensure that none of the following conditions exist. If there is any doubt whatsoever, consult your medical doctor or an experienced massage therapist.

ACUTE INFLAMMATIONS

Massage should be avoided in most cases of acute inflammatory conditions, whether it be inflammation of muscle tissue or joint as occurs immediately after a muscle tear or joint sprain; inflammation of the skin occurring, for instance, immediately after a burn; or inflammation of an internal organ such as nephritis (inflammation of a kidney).

Massage over the site of an inflammation could further inflame the injury. However, once the acute stage has passed and the initial redness and soreness has subsided, massage may be performed above and below the injury. This will assist the circulation and encourage the flow of lymph away from the area. After several treatments, the injured area itself may be massaged to prevent the formation of fibrous adhesions.

INFECTIOUS AND CONTAGIOUS DISEASES

Massage therapy is, of course, contra-indicated if the patient has any contagious or infectious disease, or if the patient has a high temperature. It is only after the infectious stage of any disease that massage therapy may be used beneficially.

PREGNANCY AND MENSTRUATION

Abdominal massage is generally contra-indicated if a woman is pregnant or menstruating because the internal organs are often tender and very active, and any deep manipulation of the tissues could cause disruption or injury. However, very gentle massage using only light effleurage movements is perfectly safe and often recommended to help ease pain and promote relaxation. Many women instinctively gently massage their own abdomen when they experience any tenderness or discomfort during menstruation.

RECENT WOUNDS OR SCAR TISSUE

Whilst massage can help scar tissue and wounds to heal and also prevent any fibrous adhesions forming, any massage should be done with extreme caution. Massaging over recent wounds or scar tissue can cause them to open and even infect the injury, as well as causing further injury beneath the wound. If, for instance, you have recently undergone surgery, remember that different operations cause varying degrees of internal and external scarring. Massage should, therefore, only be performed with your doctor's consent and preferably by an experienced therapist who will ensure that the treatment does not damage the site of the wound or cause internal injury.

Any massage should normally be delayed until the wound has begun to heal, and then commenced very gently to the areas around the wound, above and below, but *not* on the site of the wound itself. Only when the wound has fully healed can the site of the wound be treated and then only with extreme caution.

SKIN DISEASES

It should go without saying that massage is not a good idea if the patient has any sort of infectious or contagious skin complaint. Aside from the fact that the therapist may become infected, massage may aggravate the skin condition and make it much worse or spread it to non-affected areas of the patient's body.

It is true that some non-infectious skin disorders can be improved by massage therapy. For instance, eczema and psoriasis (two of the more common skin complaints) are often alleviated by very gentle massage using pure almond and vitamin E enriched vegetable oils as a base to which therapeutic essential oils of lavender or camomile are added.

But in practice, any skin condition can be aggravated by massage, and all skin complaints (including those that are non-infectious or non-contagious) should be treated with extreme caution. As a general rule, if a person has a skin disorder, massage therapy is usually best postponed and treatment only commenced once the condition has cleared. If you have a skin complaint of any kind remember to mention it to the massage therapist who will be able to advise you as to whether massage is appropriate.

THROMBOSIS AND PHLEBITIS

It is extremely dangerous and even life threatening to massage anyone who has thrombosis or phlebitis. Thrombosis is the formation of a blood clot (a thrombus) attached to the wall of an artery or vein, or lodged in an organ of the body, whereas phlebitis is the formation of a clot in a vein which causes the vein to inflame painfully. In either case, if the clot is dislodged, it could travel through the bloodstream and block a major artery causing a fatal stroke or a heart attack.

VARICOSE VEINS

Veins become varicose when the valves within the veins lose their strength and are unable to prevent the blood from flowing downwards. As a result the walls of the affected vein bulge out and the vein is visible through the skin. The condition can be very painful.

Massage therapy can help to prevent varicose veins from forming, but once formed, massage on a varicose vein is not to be advised as it may further damage the vein. However, it is sometimes helpful to massage a few inches above and then a few inches below the area (always gently and towards the heart) to assist the venous blood circulation.

8
BASIC THERAPEUTIC MASSAGE TECHNIQUES

The art of giving massage lies in knowing which part of the
hand to use and how much pressure to apply for each movement, and this can only be learned through practice.
> Dr Chandra Patel, *The Complete Guide to Stress
> Management.*

One of the wonderful things about the art of massage is that it
can be done by practically anyone, although your hands may
tire easily at first. All you require to be able to give someone a
basic massage is a suitable lubricant, a towel and a firm
comfortable surface such as a carpeted floor or bed on which
the recipient can lie. Alternatively an upright chair will suffice
for a neck and shoulder massage.

LUBRICANTS

Some form of lubrication is always advisable to ensure that the
tissues may be freely manipulated without fear of causing skin
irritation. A back massage can be turned into a torture session
within a minute or so without a lubricant. Any oil or cream
that enables the hands to glide easily, but firmly, over the skin
may be used. However, natural vegetable oils and balms are
preferable to synthetic preparations and mineral oils such
as baby oil. This is because, although the skin protects us from

external bacteria and toxins, it is a living organ and some substances do actually penetrate through the dermis layer. In fact, some medicines are given by way of plasters stuck onto the skin. Therefore it makes sense to use natural lubricants whenever possible.

TALCS

Talc is an excellent dry lubricant, ideal for massaging small areas and useful in circumstances where other lubricants are inconvenient. It enables the massage therapist's hands to move easily over the skin and prevents excessive friction. However it is advisable to use only a non-perfumed talc and preferably a medicated talc because the chemical perfumes sometimes irritate the skin.

Talcs should not be used on a hairy body as it may irritate the hair follicles and cause the skin to itch. It is also inadvisable to use talc for any facial massage as the powder may get into the eyes or nose and cause sneezing fits.

CREAMS

Natural creams tend to have therapeutic value and are therefore ideal for massage. Simple cold-pressed vegetable oils mixed with water and beeswax were the first recorded 'cold creams' developed by the Greek physician Galen in the second century AD. These were found to smooth and soften the skin as well as soothe and cool the dermis. However, creams do tend to be greasy and so it is advisable to test the cream on your own skin before using it to massage.

Once again, as with talcs, creams are not well suited to hairy bodies, and remember to stick to simple unperfumed varieties.

OILS

Oils are by far the most common form of lubricant used in massage therapy. I recommend only the purest cold-pressed, virgin vegetable or nut oils as these contain vitamins and other nutrients with enzymes which are lacking in the typical commercial organic oils or mineral oils. The Chinese massage therapists have traditionally used sesame oil in massage therapy but this has a pungent aroma.

Cold-pressed virgin olive oil may also be used, but this is a thick oil and can be a bit messy. Wheatgerm oil is also thick but high in vitamin E, a known anti-oxidant which slows the ageing process of the skin. Almond oil is an excellent base oil although this can be expensive. Other ideal lubricants for massage are grapeseed, sunflower, and safflower oils, all of which are relatively inexpensive and good carrier oils enabling aromatherapy essential oils to be mixed in easily.

AROMATHERAPY ESSENTIAL OILS

Aromatherapy essential oils are the concentrated essences taken from flowers, herbs and trees and are used to help treat a wide range of health problems including skin complaints, depression, nervous tension and insomnia. Hippocrates considered: 'The way to health is to have an aromatic bath and scented massage every day.'

Research is now indicating that these oils do have measurable therapeutic applications which affect our moods and emotions, for instance, jasmine, rose, bergamot, ylang ylang, geranium and peppermint are reported to help lift depression, and rose, lavender, rosewood and clary sage are all calming relaxants. Essential oils have also been shown to have noticeable physiological effects that can greatly enhance the benefits of massage therapy.

One example is the work of Dr Gary Schwartz, professor of psychology and psychiatry at Yale University who found that the aromas of some oils can actually reduce blood pressure. The scent of spiced apple, for instance, was found to reduce blood pressure by an average of three to five points in healthy volunteers.

Essential oils may be added to the base vegetable oil to provide additional benefits through the medicinal properties of the plants themselves. For instance, extract of lavender helps calm and soothe skin irritations and burns, marigold helps heal sores, and comfrey assists in reducing swellings. Essences may be added to the vegetable base oil when required, although it is important to use no more than five drops of an essential oil for every 10ml of vegetable oil. Stronger concentrations may cause skin irritation.

When handling essential oils it is important to ensure that an essential oil is never poured directly onto the skin; and never take them internally unless under strict medical supervision.

Apart from being used in massage, the essential oils may also be used in the home in a variety of ways:

In the bath – A few drops added to the water and mixed well can be very relaxing and therapeutic. Soak in the bath for a minimum of 10 minutes to receive the full benefit.

As a perfume – Add five drops of essential oil to 10ml of cold pressed vegetable oil and rub into skin.

As an air freshener – Sprinkle on a pot pourri or add the oil to some water and burn in an oil burner.

As an inhalation – Add a few drops to a bowl of very hot water. Cover your head with a towel, bend over the bowl and then breathe deeply.

Remember when purchasing essential oils to smell them first to ensure you like the aroma, and ask if it is pure oil or a synthetic copy. Needless to say, synthetic oils, although cheaper, do not have the same therapeutic benefits as the pure oils.

CHART OF ESSENTIAL OILS AND THEIR USES

Oil	*Effects*
Basil	Tonic, stimulant, eases fatigue
Bergamot	Anti-depressant, nervine, anti-inflammatory
Black pepper	Stimulant, warming, digestive tonic
Cajuput	Respiratory tonic, pain reducer, stimulant
Camomile	Soothing, calming, anti-inflammatory
Camphor	Decongestant
Cedarwood	Calming, harmonising
Cinnamon	Stimulant, circulatory tonic
Clary sage	Relaxant, warming, anti-spasmodic
Cypress	Astringent, anti-spasmodic, deodorant
Eucalyptus	Decongestant, anti-rheumatic
Fennel	Digestive, diuretic, menstrual regulation
Frankincense	Respiratory tonic, calming, anti-wrinkle
Geranium	Anti-depressant, antiseptic, hormone balancer
Hyssop	Respiratory tonic, eases fatigue, laxative
Jasmine	Anti-depressant, aphrodisiac
Juniper	Antiseptic, diuretic
Lavender	Calming and soothing
Lemon	Bactericide
Lemongrass	Tonic, antiseptic, bactericide
Marjoram	Sedative, anti-rheumatic
Melissa	Calming
Myrrh	Healing, rejuvenating, anti-fungal
Neroli (Orange Blossom)	Anti-depressant, aphrodisiac, cell rejuvenator
Patchouli	Anti-inflammatory, anti-fungal, healing
Peppermint	Digestive tonic, reduces fever, eases fatigue
Pine	Antiseptic, circulatory

Oil	Effects
Rose	Anti-depressant, aphrodisiac, hormone balancer
Rosemary	Stimulant, skin tonic, analgaesic
Sage	Analgaesic, tonic, diuretic
Sandalwood	Aphrodisiac, sedative, skin tonic, urinary tonic
Tagette	Anti-inflammatory, healing, rejuvenating
Thyme	Respiratory tonic, immuno-stimulant, circulatory
Tea Tree	Anti-fungal, bactericide, immuno-stimulant
Ylang Ylang	Anti-depressant, sedative, aphrodisiac

BASIC MASSAGE TECHNIQUES

There are four basic techniques used in a remedial massage and these movements, if practised correctly, are all that is required to give a complete therapeutic massage.

General Rules:
1. Always keep contact with recipient.
2. Always massage towards heart.
3. Keep all areas, other than area being massaged, covered and warm.
4. Make sure you have warm hands!
5. Create a relaxing environment.

1. Effleurage

Effleurage is the first movement applied in remedial massage. It is the stroking technique in which the palmar surface of one or both hands is used or, if the area being treated is small, the palmar surface of the thumbs or fingers. It is a rhythmic and soothing movement which helps induce relaxation and prepare the patient's muscles for deeper massage techniques.

Therapeutic effects

The effleurage massage technique has several very valuable therapeutic effects. The gentle stroking acts as a sedative to hyperactive, nervous and anxious patients, helping also to reduce high blood pressure. In my experience, where the patient does suffer from high blood pressure, just 10 minutes of effleurage is all that is needed to bring the pressure down by as much as 20 points. (However, it should be remembered that this will only be a temporary effect until the cause of the high blood pressure whether it be nervous tension at work, or arteriosclerosis – hardening of the arteries – is also tackled.)

Light effleurage movements applied to the forehead, temples and neck often relieve headaches and migraine, and when applied to the neck and back can help insomnia. In contrast to gentle effleurage, a firm, brisk effleurage acts as a stimulant, improving the flow of blood and lymph and thereby helping to cleanse the tissues. This is important when treating muscular injuries because encouraging the flow of lymph fluid ensures that any swelling is minimalised and that waste products do not accumulate around the site of the injury.

Effleurage is also useful in cases of muscle fatigue, or atrophy of tissues, and to relieve the symptoms of neuritis or neuralgia.

Contra-indications

There are times when effleurage should not be used, or used only with caution. Apart from the general conditions for which any form of massage is contra-indicated (see Chapter 9) effleurage can irritate the skin of a hairy person and create a rash. It should also never be applied, except when prescribed by a physician, over varicose veins or an area of inflammation as this may well aggravate the injury.

How to do it

The stroking motion of effleurage may be soft and light, or firm and strong, depending on whether treatment is required for the superficial or deep tissues. The hands should be relaxed so that they can mould to the contours of the area of the body being treated. Effleurage is always rhythmic and smooth, never jerky or abrupt. It should be done gently and slowly to soothe and relax the tissues, or firmly and briskly to stimulate blood flow.

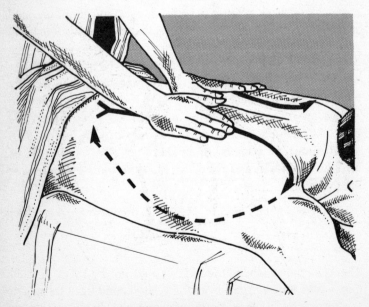

The direction of upward effleurage over the back.

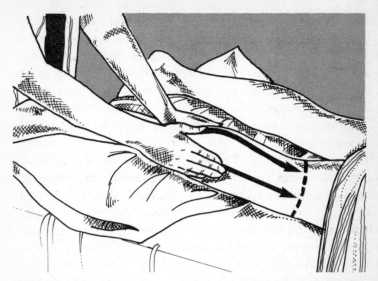

Direction of the effleurage movement over the calf muscles.

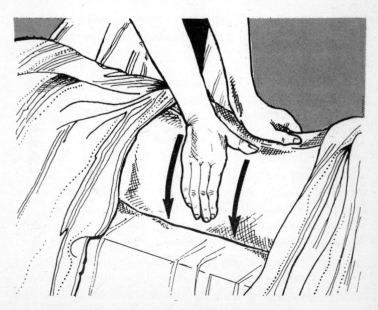

The direction of the 'lateralising' effleurage over the back.

Pressure should be applied in one direction only – usually towards the heart to assist the flow of blood through the veins back to the heart – although it is sometimes performed in a centrifugal direction (i.e. circular strokes from within, going outwards) or centripetal (i.e. circular strokes moving towards the centre). After each stroke the hands are returned to the starting point whilst lightly skimming across the skin using no pressure whatsoever. In this manner, contact is never broken between the massage therapist's hands and the patient's body, and when the effleurage movements are completed, it is easy to glide into the next technique.

2. Petrissage

Petrissage is the second technique in massage used only after the tissues have been warmed and prepared by effleurage. Petrissage derives from the word *petrir* meaning to knead and is therefore the kneading of the tissues which may be done in a variety of ways.

Therapeutic effects

The therapeutic value of petrissage is probably the most important in the field of massage. It increases circulation whilst slightly raising the temperature and helping cleanse the tissues of accumulated deposits, and it also helps improve the tone of the muscles. It is used to help break down fat deposits to be re-absorbed by the lymph, and is therefore a particularly important technique. It is often used *after* the acute phase of any injury – whether joint sprain or muscle strain – to ease the healing process by improving the blood flow to the deep tissues thereby thoroughly cleansing the muscles of accumulated metabolic wastes and by helping to strengthen the injured area.

Contra-indications

Heavy petrissage should be avoided during the acute stage of any injury as this would further inflame the injury. It should also not be applied to, or on, any *recent* scar tissue or any inflammation. It is not advisable to massage the abdomen if the patient has gastritis or colitis, and of course, deep massage should never be applied to women during pregnancy or during menstruation.

How to do it

There are several techniques employed in petrissage each to be applied in their correct sequence to achieve best results.

Picking up – The muscle is gently grasped with one or both hands and then literally picked up as if pulling the muscle away from the bone. This may be practised on the hamstrings at the back of the upper leg or the calf muscles in the lower leg. The muscle is placed between your fingers and thumb and the 'picking up' motion is created by slowly contracting the fingers

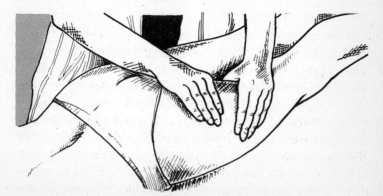

'Picking-up' over the muscles at the back of the thigh.

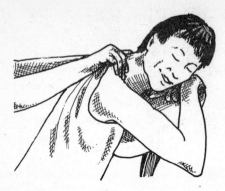

Petrissage of the trapezius region of the shoulders can be applied, as illustrated with the patient in a seated position on the plinth.

and thumb. In this movement, unlike the motion of effleurage, the fingers do not slide over the skin. A firm grasp enables the muscle to be stretched and pulled upwards away from the bone. After a few seconds the pressure is released while your hands still maintain contact with the patient.

Squeezing – Squeezing the muscle follows after the muscle has been satisfactorily loosened up by the pick up technique. The muscle is lifted exactly as before but this time, when it has been lifted it is gently squeezed in the direction of the venous blood flow (i.e. towards the heart). In this way the muscle is being cleansed of deep accumulated deposits from the tissue.

Rolling – Once the muscle has been squeezed several times and further loosened, it is then rolled transversely (i.e. across the muscle fibres) in both directions by rolling the thumb towards the fingers, and then the fingers towards the thumb. Here the thumb or fingers move smoothly over the skin but they must not merely glide, and you should be careful not to pinch the skin – the whole muscle must be lifted and rolled in the same motion.

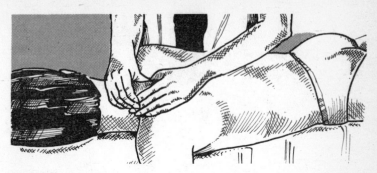

'Skin rolling' over

Wringing – The muscle is 'wrung' after having been 'rolled' which acts to separate muscle fibres and release spasms. Wringing is performed on the large muscle groups, each hand working alternately picking up the muscle between the thumb and fingers and creating a movement similar to wringing a wet towel. The action can be slow and gentle or firm and vigorous to create a relaxing or stimulating effect.

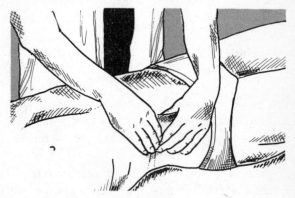

'Wringing' at the sides of the abdomen.

Kneading – Kneading is similar to wringing but works in a downward motion creating pressure rather than the lifting action of wringing and the other petrissage techniques. The hands are positioned on alternate sides of the muscle group with the hands moving in a circular motion and, as with all

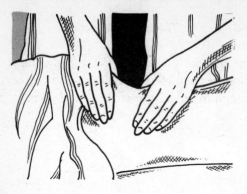

Kneading

petrissage techniques, the palms remain in full contact with the area being treated. The pressure used should start strong and lessen at the uppermost part of the circular motion, but kneading may be done slowly and gently to help relax the area being treated or firmly and briskly if stimulation is required.

3. Tapotement

Tapotement is a stimulating technique in which the muscle is pounded in a variety of ways from hacking, using the edge of the hand, to beating using the base of a fist.

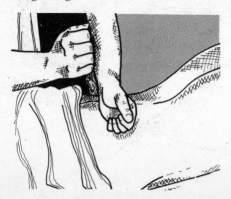

Beating

Therapeutic effects

Tapotement has the opposite effect of effleurage; it causes muscle tissue to contract and draws blood to the skin. It is therefore useful to induce muscle tone and prepare the tissues for activity.

Contra-indications

No form of tapotement should be done over the shins or other bony prominences, areas with sensitive superficial nerves (e.g. backs of knees and neck), or paralysed muscles. It should only be performed on a large muscle mass although the lighter movements may be applied to the abdomen.

How to do it

There are a variety of ways in which tapotement may be used, all of which require practice to perfect.

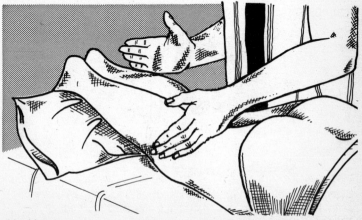

Hacking

Hacking or chopping – This is done using the outer edge of the hand much like a karate strike. Keeping the wrists very loose, the hands flick up and down very quickly and rhythmically moving only from the wrists. When seen in slow motion, the edge of the hand comes into contact with the skin first and as the movement progresses the edge of the little finger completes the movement. As the technique is learned, the hands may be turned at an angle so that the palmar surfaces are facing slightly upward which enables both hands to hit the same point on the body.

Flicking – Flicking is similar to hacking except that in the flicking movement only the edges of the little fingers and not the edge of the hand come into contact with the patient. This produces a much softer effect, stimulating the superficial tissues rather than the deep muscles.

Clapping – Clapping is done with the palms forming a hollow curve with the fingers and produces a hollow sound as opposed to a slapping sound which occurs if the hand and fingers are not rounded. It is easy to tell if it is being done correctly by listening to the action. Clapping does not hurt, slapping stings.

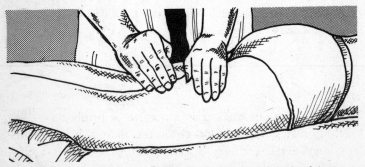

Clapping. Note how close the hands are kept to the body of the patient in both clapping and hacking. In the case of clapping, the hands are cupped and not flat.

Pounding – Pounding is done using the underside of a closed fist but the fists should be clenched yet relaxed to produce a deep yet unabrasive effect on the tissues.

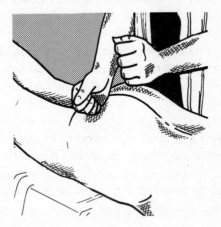

Pounding

4. Friction

Friction is created by a firm, rapid movement of the massage therapist's hand against the patient's body. Whilst this will cause a redness in the skin from the increased blood flow, it should not cause undue skin irritation.

Therapeutic effects

There are occasions when tissues need to be firmly rubbed to break up adhesions or to loosen fibrous matter. It is particularly useful in the treatment of joint disorders because it significantly increases blood flow to the area.

Contra-indications

Friction is inappropriate if the skin is delicate or sensitive as it could well irritate it. It is also not advisable to use the friction technique on or near the site of a recent wound because it could cause further injury. Remember any massage movement should be deliberate and controlled and there is a danger with friction that the control is lost.

How to do it

Friction is most effectively done using the palmar surface of the thumb, fingers or side of the hand depending upon the size of the area being treated. It is created by pressing down firmly and simultaneously rubbing to induce heat and increase circulation to the area. This needs to be done quickly but with sufficient lubrication to prevent skin irritation.

Combining the techniques

The massage techniques should be combined in a specific sequence to obtain maximum benefit. In fact, I would go even further by saying that if the sequence is disturbed, it could actually make the person's condition worse. For instance, a strained muscle should be relaxed with effleurage before it is kneaded with petrissage because immediate petrissage could further damage the injured muscle fibres.

Always begin relaxing the muscles by effleurage, and only then move on to petrissage to begin cleansing the tissues of metabolic wastes. This may be followed by friction if required (e.g. around a joint), in which case it should be petrissaged once again. Only then is any tapotement appropriate, and this will be in limited circumstances, before returning to finish the treatment with effleurage.

It is also important to remember that at no time during the treatment should the hands of the massage therapist leave the recipient's body. This is principally to keep the sensory nerves stimulated and thereby maintain the physical relaxation of the muscle being treated as well as the mental relaxation of the person being massaged. Any break of contact interrupts the rhythm of the treatment.

Always massage above the area being treated before massaging lower down. For instance, massage above the knee before concentrating on the area below the knee so that the lymph can be cleared efficiently.

9
SELF-MASSAGE

Therapeutic massage is something everyone can do for themselves albeit to a limited degree. There are of course obvious limitations – it is difficult to relax and massage at the same time, and it is not easy to massage your own back – and massaging yourself is by no means as effective or beneficial as having a proper massage from a qualified massage therapist. But there are many ways self-massage can be done, and is done often instinctively, to help relieve a variety of minor everyday health problems. You only have to remember the last time you banged your elbow to realise how you first relieved the pain.

The wonderful thing about self-massage is that it is such a simple therapy it needs no more than your hands, and it can be done with great effect wherever you happen to be – in the office, the home, or even when travelling in a car, train or aeroplane. Below is a list of common everyday ailments that respond well to self-massage, with a brief description of how to do the appropriate massage technique. Whilst all techniques are perfectly safe and have no side effects, in all cases it is advisable to consult your doctor or massage therapist before commencing any self-treatment.

BACKACHE

Lie on a firm base (e.g. a carpeted floor) face upwards, pull your knees to your chest and gently rock forwards and backwards for 60 seconds. This massages the spine and frees minor restrictions in the facet joints of the vertebrae.

Sit up, putting your hands behind your back, press your fingers firmly into the top of the buttocks and push sharply four times. Repeat all around the top of the buttocks starting in the middle and working outwards, and then do exactly the same either side of the lumbar (lower) spine.

Backache — 2nd exercise

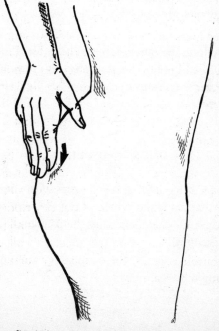

Press fingers firmly into the top of the buttocks and push sharply 4 times.

Backache — 3rd exercise

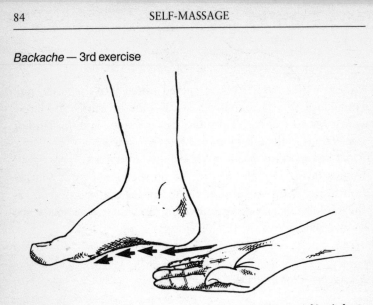

Palm of hand or thumb presses firmly against the instep of both feet.

Press firmly along the inner arches of both feet moving from the ankle up to the big toe. This is a reflexology technique that stimulates the nerve endings and creates a reflex effect in the back.

COLDS AND FLU

Thump the centre of your chest seven times with your fist. This stimulates the thymus gland which is now known to activate the body's immune system and also helps loosen up mucus congestion in the lungs.

CONSTIPATION

Gently massage your abdomen pressing firmly with both hands, one on top of the other. Beginning on the lower right

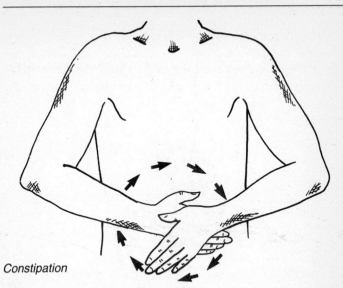

Constipation

hand side and moving your hands in a circular motion, massage up towards the ribs, across to the left side, downwards, and then back across to the right. Continue this movement for five to ten minutes morning and evening.

CRAMP

Stretch the affected muscle group and follow by gentle, yet firm, stroking movements which will help relax the muscles and thus relieve the pain. (Rubbing the centre of the muscle with a piece of copper often brings immediate relief.)

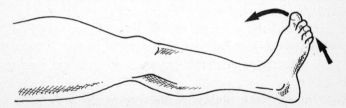

Gently stretch the muscle and then lightly massage up the leg.

EYE STRAIN

Rest your head in the palms of your hands, gently pressing the palms into the eye sockets, then move your palms in a circular motion to the left and then to the right. Continue for up to five minutes.

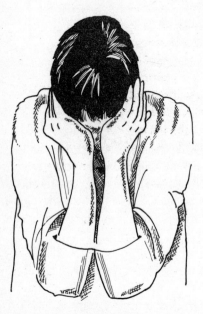

Massage eyes with the palms of the hands.

HEADACHES

Press firmly with the index and middle finger of each hand into the bottom of the occipital bone at the base of the head (where the skull joins the spine). Hold for seven seconds and repeat three times.

Press firmly using the index and middle fingers on the temple and make circular movements in both directions.

Headaches

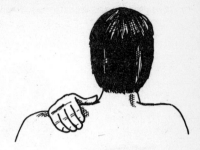

(A)
Press fingers into base
of the head at the back.

(B)
Base of head

Rub temples in a circular motion
using index and middle fingers.

TENSION IN NECK AND SHOULDERS

Press the fingers of your right hand into the right side of the
base of the head, and the fingers of the left hand into the left
side. Hold the pressure for seven seconds and repeat three times.

Tension in Neck and Shoulders

1. As in (A) above

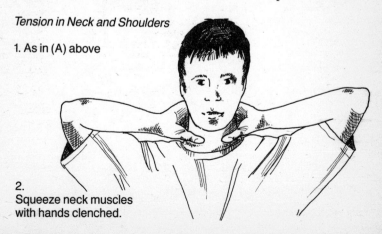

2.
Squeeze neck muscles
with hands clenched.

Fold your hands behind your neck, and using your thumbs, squeeze the muscles together. Slowly work your way up to the top of the neck.

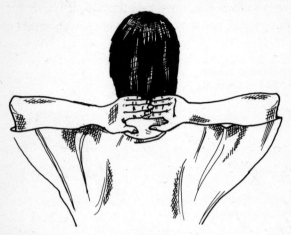

Using your right hand, squeeze the neck and shoulder muscles on the left side and repeat using the left hand on the right side.

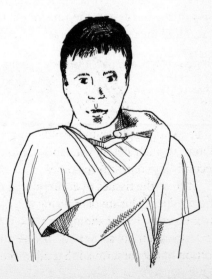

3.
Using right hand squeeze left side of the neck and shoulders.

TENNIS ELBOW

It is imperative that you consult a qualified practitioner if you have tennis elbow but, if you feel the muscles in your forearms becoming tense, you may be able to prevent the onset of tennis elbow.

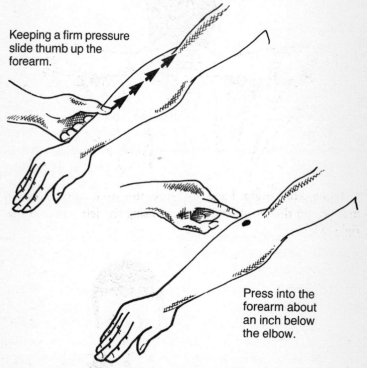

Keeping a firm pressure slide thumb up the forearm.

Press into the forearm about an inch below the elbow.

Press your right thumb firmly into the top of the left forearm about an inch below the elbow. Hold the pressure for seven seconds and repeat three times.

Cleanse the tissues of accumulated deposits by stripping out the muscles. This involves using the right thumb to maintain a firm pressure whilst sliding up the left forearm. Use some form of lubrication so as not to irritate the skin and repeat each section of the forearm so that all of the muscle is covered.

10
CHINESE MASSAGE THERAPY

It is my feeling that the clinical work in massage therapy done in China is without equal in the world. The extremely effective work in this modality follows from the over three millenia of experience in traditional Chinese medicine.

Dr Ronald Puhky,
Bachelor of Acupuncture,
College of Traditional Medicine UK.

Therapeutic massage has a long tradition in Chinese medical literature and dates back to the *Nei Ching* reputed to be over 4000 years old. In fact, it was Chinese massage therapy that first inspired Professor Ling, during his travels, to experiment with massage in Europe.

However, traditional Chinese medicine does not place paramount importance on the human anatomy and physiology as we in the West understand it. Instead, the Chinese physicians concentrate on channels of energy – known as 'meridians' – which are believed to travel along particular paths and in specific directions in the body.

Until recently these meridians were dismissed by conventional Western medicine as nonsense despite the overwhelming historical and empirical evidence in support of the Chinese theory. After all, Chinese surgeons have been performing standard surgical operations for years without any chemical anaesthetics but instead were using only acupuncture needles which pierce the skin at specific points along the meridians. Recent studies conducted by the British Medical Association acknowledged that the system of acupuncture does, at the very least, affect the production of endorphines and encephalins in the brain, and it has long been known that these chemicals relieve pain and help in the treatment of disease.

The other fundamental tenet of Chinese medical philosophy is the principle of yin and yang which, in essence, expresses balance. The universe is said to consist of opposing forces which are balanced in nature. Dark and light, dry and wet, cold and hot, are examples of these forces which are as different as night from day and yet together they produce harmony. The whole of nature depends upon the balancing of the yin qualities with the yang, and it is only when there is an imbalance that disorder sets in. Likewise the human body has yin and yang qualities. At any one time the body, or part of it, may be too cold or too hot, too dry or too wet, too active or too passive. A Chinese physician examines a patient with the yin and yang principle and the body's energies in mind, and the selected treatment will aim to restore and maintain balance.

The Chinese system of massage therapy, like all traditional Chinese medicine, focuses on balancing the yin qualities with the yang and influencing the energy channels in the human body. A system was devised called 'acupressure' (pressure of a point) which identifies the same points as those used in acupuncture. Healing is promoted by stimulating the flow of energy through the meridians as well as releasing tension and improving blood circulation. The fundamental difference between this method and acupuncture is that the massage therapist does not insert needles, but instead uses the gentle but firm pressure of his fingers, hands, elbows, knees and even feet on the patient's body.

Despite the fact that there are, today, more sophisticated methods of stimulating the acupoints using electrical devices –

and, of course, needles – acupressure continues to be widely used and has been shown to be the most effective in the relief of stress-related ailments and in preventive health care.

The Handbook of Chinese Massage Therapy compiled at the Anhui Medical School Hospital in China and published in 1983 states:

> There is extensive scope for the application of massage therapy. It can be used for numerous diseases in the fields of internal, surgical, paediatric and traumatic medicine. Generally speaking, massage therapy is suitable for chronic and functional diseases. However, it can also have a good therapeutic effect in certain acute illnesses, such as the common cold, acute sprains, etc. The traumatic conditions it is most used in include acute sprain, contusion, chronic strain, a lumbar slipped intervertebral disc and fractures of the limbs. The internal diseases it is most used in are the common cold, acute gastro-enteritis, ulcers, gastroptosis, paralysis, and rheumatoid arthritis. The paediatric diseases where massage therapy is most frequently used are acute upper respiratory tract infections, digestive disturbances, chronic nutritional disturbances, and poliomyelitis.

Reading the above text, it soon becomes obvious that massage therapy is a well-respected and well-practised medicine in China even to this day. There are over 40 massage techniques used to stimulate the internal organs as well as to stimulate or sedate the nerves, relax the muscles, and improve blood flow and lymph drainage.

However, as the Eastern and Western systems of massage therapy develop, it is interesting to note the growing similarities in practice. For instance, the trigger points used by Western massage therapists to affect a muscle group or indeed an internal organ generally fall on what are called the 'origin and insertion' points. These are the points at which the muscle is connected to the tendon (which attaches to the bone), and analysis of the Chinese meridians reveals that many of the acupoints lie on exactly the same origin and insertion points.

Like Western massage therapy, the Chinese use differing forms of lubrication although less of it as they tend to use more friction in a typical treatment. Fresh ginger juice is the most common form of lubricant, especially in the treatment of children, because the juice is very slippery and enables the massage therapist's hands to glide easily without excessive friction to the child's delicate skin. It also has the added benefit of producing a radiating warmth when applied.

Sesame oil is the usual oil prescribed, and occasionally cinnamon oil to produce a fragrant heat. Talc is sometimes used as a mild lubricant for treatment on small areas, but the therapist may also use a strong alcohol (typically 65 per cent proof) to help lower the temperature of a patient suffering with a fever, or egg white for abdominal massage, as well as numerous Chinese herbal compounds.

THE 10 MINUTE CHINESE ENERGY MASSAGE

The 10 minute Chinese Energy Massage is a quick, easy-to-learn system of massage which stimulates the main energy channels and affects all of the major organs in the body. It releases tremendous energies, leaving the patient feeling calm yet invigorated. It is commonly used, not only as a general tonic to maintain good health, but also to help patients suffering from fatigue or recovering from illness. However, if you are suffering from any spinal disorder, disease or deformity it is always advisable to consult your doctor before commencing this massage. The energy massage is very easy to perform. It is a simple back massage and can be performed at any time of day. There are three steps in the massage: preparation, stimulation and finally sedation, all of which must be done in their correct sequence.

The preparation stage begins by removing blockages in the energy channels, the stimulation stage stimulates the energy flows, and the sedatory stage calms and soothes the energies.

It is very important to massage in the correct direction, i.e. to follow the flow of energy – in this instance, it is always up the spine and down the sides of the back. There is also one other important point to remember: all three stages should be done in repetitions of three.

The energy massage is best done with a vegetable oil base mixed with the essential oils of myrrh, neroli and geranium although other essential oils may also be used.

The massage begins with effleurage (gentle stroking) and ends with effleurage, and in between each stage continuity is maintained using the same light effleurage.

THE PREPARATION STAGE

The preparation stage uses both thumbs alternately; as one slides, the other releases so that each thumb massages a small section of the spine before the other thumb is used. Keeping a firm pressure, and using short movements, move up the spine pressing on the vertebrae in one line towards the base of the neck. Then, using the same movements, return in two columns (approximately 1½ inches and 3 inches apart and to the right of the spine) down the right side of the back. Then up the spine again, and down the left side. Repeat this sequence three times, then follow it with light effleurage, again up the spine and down the sides before moving on to the second stage.

THE STIMULATION STAGE

For this stage a 'hacking' or 'chopping' movement is used and, like the effleurage, is done up the spine and down the sides of

CHINESE MASSAGE

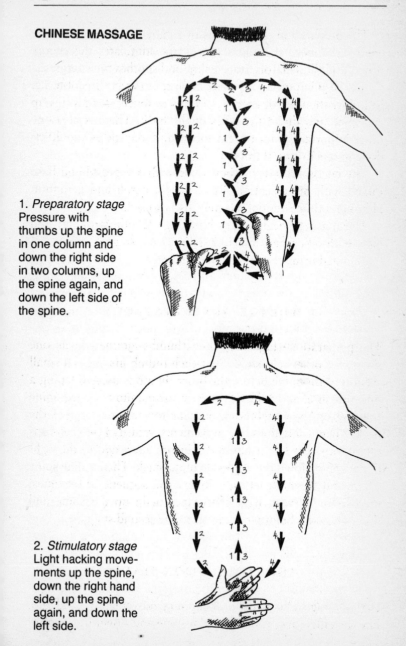

1. *Preparatory stage* Pressure with thumbs up the spine in one column and down the right side in two columns, up the spine again, and down the left side of the spine.

2. *Stimulatory stage* Light hacking movements up the spine, down the right hand side, up the spine again, and down the left side.

the back. With the hands held perpendicular to the spine, move up the spine using very light hacking movements and making sure you hit the depression between the vertebrae which is where the acupoints are situated. Try to keep the fingers close together as this way you will be sure to hit every acupoint. Then return down the right side of the back, before going back up the spine and then down the left side. Repeat this sequence three times and then, once again, do three more effleurage movements before proceeding to the third and final stage.

THE SEDATORY STAGE

This is done with the palmar surfaces of both hands, one palm down on top of the other. Slowly, firmly and deliberately slide the hands up the spine. If you need to exert more pressure, stand on one foot and put most of your body weight on to the hands. On reaching the base of the neck, separate your hands and let them gently slide down either side of the spine. Repeat this three times and then begin one more slide upwards. As you reach the neck, massage the neck and shoulders by placing the fingers over the shoulders leaving the thumbs at the nape of the neck and use the thumbs to massage the neck and shoulder muscles. Move the thumbs in slow, circular movements, moving from the base of the neck to the top of the shoulders and back again three times.

End the massage with gentle pressure to the spine using both hands, one on top of the other as above, moving from the base of the spine up to the neck as before, and then softly bringing the hands down the sides of the back.

Finally, wipe off any excess oil with a paper towel moving in the same direction as used in the massage – up the spine and down the sides.

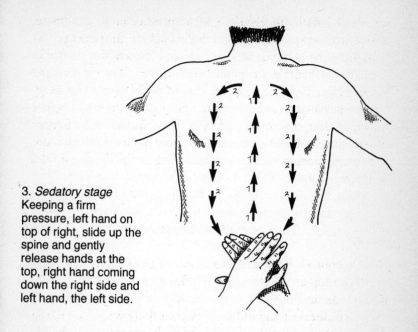

3. *Sedatory stage*
Keeping a firm
pressure, left hand on
top of right, slide up the
spine and gently
release hands at the
top, right hand coming
down the right side and
left hand, the left side.

THE CHINESE SELF-MASSAGE FOR STRENGTHENING THE BODY AND PREVENTING ILL-HEALTH

The Chinese self-massage takes only 10–15 minutes to do and completely invigorates the body by stimulating the energy channels. It is best done first thing in the morning and in the open air if possible. Repeat each movement at least three times, and seven times if possible.

- Shake the arms, wrists, legs and ankles vigorously.
- Jump up and down from one foot to the other, relaxing the shoulders so that the arms hang loose.
- Rub both hands together rapidly until they are warm.

- Make loose fists and tap all over the head and down the sides and back of the neck.
- Tilt the head back and gently squeeze the back of the neck with one hand and then the other.
- Rub the forehead with the three middle finger tips in a circular motion.
- Pinch the eyebrows with the thumb and index finger starting from the centre and working towards the outside of the brows.
- Gently massage the eyelids and below the eye sockets.
- Using the side of the index finger, rub up and down the side of the nose vigorously, whilst breathing deeply.
- Using the thumbs or finger tips, massage:
  1. upper and lower gums
  2. under the cheek bones
  3. under the jaw bone to the back of the ears
- Rotate, pull and flick off the top of the ears, then the middle of the ears, and finally the ear lobes.
- Slide the hands firmly above the ears towards the back of the head.
- Hold out the left arm, support it at the elbow with the right hand, and with a loose fist tap:
  1. the right shoulder
  2. down the inside of the right arm
  3. up the outside of the right arm

Then stretch the wrist, rotate the thumb and fingers, before shaking the right arm.

Repeat the process on the left arm.

- Bend forward, and with knees bent and a loose fist:
  1. tap down each side of the spine
  2. tap on the base of the spine
  3. tap buttocks
  4. tap down the outside of the legs
  5. tap up the insides of the legs
- Massage the abdomen, pressing gently but firmly, and

moving in a clockwise direction up the right side of the abdomen to the rib cage, across, and down the left side following the colon.

Finish off by shaking the whole of your body thoroughly, and you will feel completely energised.

11
MASSAGE THERAPY IN SPORT

Massage is one of the basics of training that somehow got lost. I know that without it I would be injured much more than I am now.

Mary Decker Slaney, Olympic athlete.

Massage is the oldest form of sports medicine, traceable as far back as the Olympic games of ancient Greece. Yet it is only in recent years that massage has once again begun to be used in the treatment and prevention of sports-related injuries. Sports men and women are experiencing for themselves the benefits of incorporating massage therapy into their programmes.

Athletes and sports' doctors, two visible and well-respected groups, began speaking up for massage therapy in sports medicine several years ago, and there is little doubt that massage has received a tremendous boost from the endorsement of sports figures such as runners Rob de Castella, Joan Benoit, Mary Decker Slaney, Lasse Virren and Charlie Spedding, as well as the British Olympic cycling team, the Amateur Athletics Association and the Football Association. The New York Giants American football team also use the services of a massage therapist.

THE BENEFITS OF MASSAGE IN SPORT

Massage has special benefits for all sports men and women. Athletes use it to improve circulation and reduce nervous tension before an event, and to relieve tightness in the muscles. Runners and footballers use it to warm muscles making them more flexible and helping to prevent tears in the tissues, rugby players require massage to promote healing of bruises, muscle strains and joint sprains, and many sports men and women have massage therapy simply to help reduce nervous tension and to relax the mind before an important event.

But where massage comes into its own in sports therapies is in its ability to help cleanse the tissues and keep the muscles free from any restrictions. Massage encourages the body to remove lactic acid (a metabolic waste product of muscle movement) from fatigued muscles after the event. Ben Benjamin Ph.D, sports medicine specialist and founder of the Muscular Therapy Institute in Cambridge, Massachusetts has said: 'Lactic acid build-up can occur during exercise, causing muscle cramps. Massage really helps reduce pain and fatigue.'

When muscles are exercised, chemical waste products including lactic acid and urea are released into the muscles and these may then crystallise causing cramps, stiffness and pain. It is these waste products that often cause muscles to ache and feel sore a day or so after rigorous exercise. Massage helps prevent these accumulations forming in the muscles by helping to speed up their elimination from the tissues.

The Football Association Guide to the Treatment and Rehabilitation of Injuries in Sport (Heinemann 1983) refers to massage therapy used on injured soccer players and summarises the benefits as follows:

a. Massage stimulates circulation, shifts exudate and remobilises tissues that have been bound by scarring and adhesions.

b. Massage is a great help in pre-season training and as an anti-fatigue measure after the match. It rapidly reduces stiffness and soreness and is excellent for finding local sore spots for further diagnosis and treatment.

Sports massage is an extension of basic massage with additional special techniques to help alleviate specific injuries to the muscles and tendons, thereby promoting recovery from muscle injury and/or fatigue. Unlike basic massage, sports massage is primarily designed to invigorate rather than relax and therefore differs quite considerably in approach and techniques used from general massage.

HOW MASSAGE IS USED IN SPORT

There are four types of sports massage: pre-event massage, post-event massage, inter-competition massage, and clinical sports massage.

PRE-EVENT MASSAGE

Pre-event massage is invigorating; its function is to prepare muscles for work and make sure they are sufficiently flexible to maximise performance and minimise the possibility of muscle strain during the event. Muscles need to be loose and warm before any hard physical exercise so that you can move quickly, stretch, twist and turn as required by the demands of the sport. A pre-event massage is a short treatment usually lasting anywhere between five minutes and half-an-hour, in which the muscles are pummelled using fast, vigorous movements to activate the muscles and stimulate circulation.

POST-EVENT MASSAGE

Post-event massage is specifically designed to help your muscles recover from fatigue. It is a slow, yet firm, massage which gently relaxes the muscles, and focuses on cleansing the tissues of lactic acids and other deposits to encourage a fast and efficient recovery. Top athletes use massage therapy to speed up recovery from training and competition events, and have been able to narrow their recovery time, in some instances, from three to four days to only one day.

INTER-COMPETITION MASSAGE

Inter-competition massage is performed during breaks in activity between successive events and is, as you might expect, a combination of pre- and post-event therapy. It promotes fast recovery of the muscles after one event and then goes on to invigorate the muscles preparing them for the next event. The inter-competition massage is mostly used at events held over a short space of time – one-day competitions, athletics meetings, tennis tournaments, swimming galas, as well as the inter-national world cups, and Olympic games.

CLINICAL SPORTS MASSAGE

Clinical sports massage is perhaps the most important treatment for the professional sports person and those sports men and women who take their sport seriously. For a start, regular contact with a massage therapist helps the sports person maintain motivation and enthusiasm for training. But, more importantly, clinical sports massage helps to identify muscular strengths and weaknesses and points to problem areas in muscles before they become major injuries. It is, therefore, primarily preventive sports medicine.

Clinical sports massage also provides a good indicator as to whether the athlete is training too hard or not hard enough. Frequent soreness and stiffness in the muscles may indicate that the training programme is too severe, whereas flaccid, loose muscles may indicate that more rigorous training is necessary.

Pre-event massage, post-event massage and inter-competition massage all usually take place on the day of the sporting event and at the sports ground itself, and the typical treatment time is between five minutes to half-an-hour depending upon the area of the body requiring treatment. A clinical sports massage, on the other hand, is usually only done in a clinical environment and the treatment time is between 45 minutes and an hour.

A massage therapist can help you schedule your massage sessions after he or she has reviewed your training schedule and (when applicable) your competition schedule.

MASSAGE AND SPORTS PERFORMANCE

Although there's no conclusive evidence that massage can improve athletic performance, many athletes swear by it. Sprinters feel that they can run faster, marathon runners have more stamina, cyclists seem to have more power in their legs, and squash players feel more agile. Football and rugby players say they feel stronger and fitter when having regular massage.

Massage has been used for many years now at numerous competitions to help competitors reduce the recovery time between events. The British Olympic cycling team took two massage therapists along with them to the 1988 games in Seoul; the Amateur Athletics Association funded a massage therapist to attend world cup mountain races in France, and in North America, 14 massage therapists were working at the

Western Canadian Summer Games in 1988 and 1989. Today, many Olympic teams sponsor their own massage therapists and have them on hand at the event.

Cyclist Greg LeMond had the help of a massage therapist for his three Tour de France wins. Rob de Castella, an international long-distance runner who has competed in the marathon event at several Olympic games, attributed much of his success to his sports massage. 'Sometimes my legs were so sore that Royce [his massage therapist] could barely work with them,' de Castella said. 'But he always loosened them up in the end.' Partially as a result of this therapy, de Castella was placed eighth in the Seoul Olympics. His performance made him the first runner ever to finish in the top 10 of three consecutive Olympic marathons – testimony to the effectiveness of regular massage therapy.

Since Rob de Castella discovered massage therapy in 1983, he always travels to important races with a therapist. 'The Australian team didn't have a masseur back in 1984 before the Los Angeles Games, so I found my own,' he said. Nowadays, the Australian national team, perhaps having learned something from de Castella, also travels with a massage therapist.

Experiences such as these seem to be validated by a small study from Sweden. Eight competitive cyclists pedalled to exhaustion, then were tested for muscle strength under two conditions: after one set of rides, the cyclists rested for 10 minutes; after another, they received a 10-minute massage. Their leg strength after massage was 11 per cent greater than after the rest period.

Sports massage has become one of the fastest expanding forms of preventive and remedial therapies in sports medicine. Sports massage therapists, long relied upon in Europe in gruelling events like multi-day cycle races, have recently begun to enjoy more esteem in the United States. The University of Texas women's track team, for example, employs a full-time therapist. At major triathlons, the top finishers dash into the massage tent as soon as they complete the race. And massage tents have been popping up at the biggest road races, particularly marathons.

Mexico's Arturo Barrios, world record holder for 10,000 metres, likes to get a massage at least once a week. 'Whenever I race, it usually takes me two or three days to recover,' he says. 'But if I get a massage right away, it only takes 24 hours to feel better.'

'But I don't just get massage after races, when I do a long run on the Switzerland Trail [a rocky trail above Boulder, where Barrios lives], my legs get beat up, so I go for a massage. I can feel the difference right away.'

MASSAGE AND TRAINING

Though many are still just learning about the benefits of massage, more and more sports men and women are using massage to enhance their training and help solve muscle problems. 'We don't diagnose or prescribe,' says Gene Arbetter of the American Massage Therapy Association, 'but we can help runners move in a pain-free manner. Our work is results-oriented.'

It goes without saying, of course, that massage alone can't make you a better athlete. While it can assist you in reaching peak form, it can't do the hard work and training for you. That's why Ingrid Kristiansen says she likes massage but doesn't depend on it. 'Massage is good if you have soreness or an injury,' she says, 'but it is not the same as hard training.' But with healthy, well-maintained muscles, you can train harder and improve your racing. Vicki Ash, a 2:49 marathoner from Boulder, USA, said regular massage therapy led to her improvement. Before beginning massage, Ash was able to train only 30 to 40 miles a week. Regular massage enabled her to build her workout schedule to the point where she qualified for the 1988 US Olympic Marathon Trials.

Ultimately, you don't have to be fine-tuning your body in preparation for an Olympic event to benefit from massage therapy. For whatever sport you may do, massage will improve your training, encourage fast recovery from fatigue and injury, and also help prevent your injuries. The last word I will leave to Mary Decker Slaney:

> 'I recommend massage to athletes at any level of ability, from world class to weekend competition. It will not only improve your performance, it will speed your recovery time and cut down on the number of muscle injuries. And all of that will make sport more fun, which is really what it is all about anyway.'

MASSAGE AND COMMON SPORTS INJURIES

Massage is one of the most effective remedial treatments for sports injuries because it treats the muscles, tendons and ligaments – the very tissues damaged in most sports injuries. Massage therapy is vastly superior to most other treatments because it works with the body's own healing processes by improving circulation to and from the injured tissues and thereby helps to prevent the formation of adhesions or scar tissue. It is also an excellent preventive therapy because regular treatment helps keep the tissues balanced, flexible, and free from adhesions (knotted muscle fibres).

Most general practitioners do not have a great deal of time or sympathy for sports-related injuries as they regard them as self inflicted. Consequently many patients rarely get a thorough examination or effective treatment. In fact, in my experience, most amateur sports enthusiasts who consult their doctor concerning a sports injury receive a cursory glance and are prescribed analgaesics (pain-killing drugs) and/or anti-inflammatory medications. The problem with this sympto-matic treatment is that whilst it often relieves pain in the short-term, it can help create more serious long-term problems.

Pain-killing drugs and anti-inflammatory medications do nothing to help repair the damaged tissues and, because the pain has been temporarily alleviated, many people actually unwittingly worsen the condition by using the injured muscles when they should be resting. Pain is the body's way of forcing us to rest and seek help. Masking over the pain simply enables you to further damage the tissues.

Massage tackles the problems head-on, directly treating the damaged tissues which cause the pain. Treatment often includes cryopathy (ice therapy) to help reduce inflammations and infra-red treatment (heat rays) used to warm deep muscle tissues. I have listed below a few of the more common injuries that respond very well to massage therapy giving where appro-priate the typical time scale for recovery. Please bear in mind that these time estimates are only approximations. We all heal at different rates depending upon our lifestyle. For instance, someone who smokes and drinks excessive amounts of alcohol (i.e. over 4 units per week) will recover at a much slower rate than non-smokers and teetotallers.

Most sports enthusiasts, amateur and professional, are eager to get back to their sport and often this over zealousness causes a recurrence of the problem due to the injury not having had adequate time to heal. The experienced massage therapist needs to monitor the injury regularly to be able to advise when the sport may be resumed and whether any temporary supports or other aids will be necessary.

SPORTS FIRST AID

The critical time in the onset of all sports injuries is the first 24 hours. It is this time that determines how the injury will develop and how quickly a person will recover. There are simple measures that can be taken to help the body's healing processes after an injury. The easy way to remember what to do in all cases of muscular injury is to keep the word RICE in your mind.

R = rest. Rest the injured limb or area. Take all pressure and strain off the area to allow the body's healing process to work as efficiently as possible. Further strain leads to further pain, and worsens the original damage.

I = ice. Ice packs (a packet of frozen peas will do the job nicely) should be placed on the injured area for 10–15 minutes when it is angry and inflamed, and repeated every 4–5 hours. If there is no redness, you can substitute the ice packs with hot and cold packs (hot-water bottle and an ice pack) – hot for three minutes followed by cold for one minute, repeated two or three times. This will increase blood and lymph flow to the area; increase the number of white blood cells and metabolism in the area; and help prevent adhesions forming (fibres sticking together), all thereby stimulating the healing process.

C = compression. Wrap the area in a bandage to prevent further swelling. The bandage should not be so tight as to cause pain; remember, the swelling is the body's natural reaction and part of the healing process, directing blood fluids and lymph to the injured area to bathe and nourish it. But our sedentary lifestyle encourages the body to over-compensate, and the larger the swelling, the longer it will take for the area to get back to its original state.

E = elevation. Keep the limb or area elevated to allow easy flow of blood and lymph away from the area. In many cases poor circulation is the cause of the formation of adhesions; the lymph becomes sticky and then hardens, joining muscular fibres together. Once adhesions are formed they have to be broken down and this can take months.

In all sports activities it is important to take the time beforehand to warm up properly and stretch the muscles to help prevent the possibility of straining or tearing the tissues. Similarly, after the sport it is important to finish with light exercise to wind down and then re-stretch the muscles as this helps to minimise metabolic waste products depositing in the tissues and thereby prevent the muscles seizing up.

TENNIS ELBOW

Tennis elbow is a slight misnomer because although the elbow is the site of the pain, the condition is actually caused by the forearm extensor muscles becoming inflamed due to continuous strain. It can be an extremely painful condition affecting the lateral side of the elbow which has been known, in some cases, to cause excruciating pain even when attempting a relatively small task such as picking up a cup of tea.

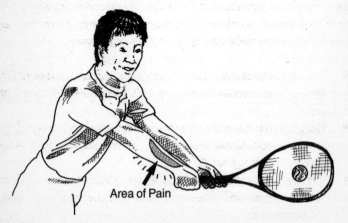

Area of Pain

Tennis Elbow

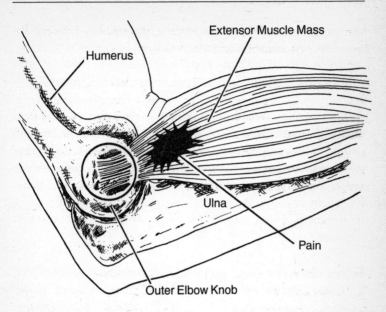

Tennis Elbow

Most tennis players usually suffer it to some degree during their lives because the holding and swinging a tennis racquet puts excessive strain on the forearm muscles, especially if the tennis racquet is too heavy or the grip too large. Nevertheless, it is easily prevented by taking simple precautions:

- It is important to select your tennis racquet carefully to ensure that it is the right weight and the handle the correct size.
- Before playing tennis, warm up the muscles by shaking the arms vigorously and massaging a warm liniment into them and then gently stretch them.
- When playing tennis, remember to give the arm a rest in between points by holding your racquet in your non-playing hand.
- Do not play for long periods of time (i.e. over an hour)

especially if you have not played during the last few weeks. The muscles will be weak and need strengthening before they will be able to cope with longer periods of play without straining.

At the first sign of tenderness or pain in the forearm, treatment should be immediately sought because, if it is left, the tendons can become irritated and, over a period of time, calcification (lime salt deposits) occurs to the tendon fibres which often require surgery. It is a condition that requires rest and remedial treatment and it responds well to massage particularly when treatment is given within 48 hours of the symptoms first occurring.

GOLFER'S ELBOW

Golfer's elbow is very similar to tennis elbow except that it affects the medial side of the elbow caused by the straining of the forearm flexor muscles. It is less common than tennis elbow because the golf club is lighter than a tennis racquet and a golfer has to rest his arm in between swings whilst he walks to his next shot. It commonly occurs when a player spends time at a driving range, hitting shot after shot.

It is easily treated by massage but requires rest and then strengthening exercises to help prevent it recurring. As with tennis elbow, to prevent it occurring, you need only take sensible precautions:

- Do not spend over one hour at a driving range if you have not been for several weeks and do not do continuous drives without breaking for a rest every half hour.
- Strengthen the forearm muscles with regular exercise.
- Have a massage treatment at least once a month to keep the muscles balanced and free from acid deposits.

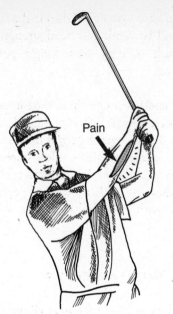

Golfer's Elbow

FOOTBALLER'S GROIN STRAIN

Hardly a week goes by in the football season when I am not consulted by someone with a groin strain. It occurs mostly at the beginning of a game after a player attempts a big kick. The muscles and tendons in the groin tear or strain largely because the player has not warmed up properly or is simply unfit.

Massage therapy is very effective in the treatment of most groin strains because it helps prevent the formation of adhesions or scar tissue and encourages the body's healing process by improving blood flow to and from the site of the injury. It usually takes between 3 weeks and 3 months to recover from a typical groin strain. However, there are occasions when a strong tackle will cause a violent impact in the groin which rips the muscles and, in these cases, surgery may be required and

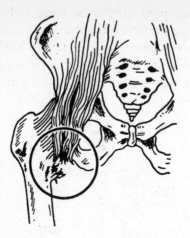

Footballer's Groin Strain

the injured player may not be able to play football for 6 months to a year.

Most groin strains may be avoided by taking the following preventive measures:

- Warm up thoroughly before playing, using a strong liniment massaged into the muscles followed by gentle stretches and light jogging.
- Exercise regularly to maintain general fitness
- Have a massage treatment at least once a month to keep the muscles flexible and free from accumulated acid deposits.

SPRINTERS' HAMSTRING

A pulled hamstring is a common sports injury particularly amongst sprinters and is usually caused by over training or poor fitness. The hamstrings are put under tremendous pressure when we sprint and this can result in the muscle fibres being suddenly torn or badly strained.

In all cases the sprinter is trying to run harder and faster than the hamstring muscles are able to go and experiences a sudden stabbing pain in the back of the leg accompanied by muscle weakness.

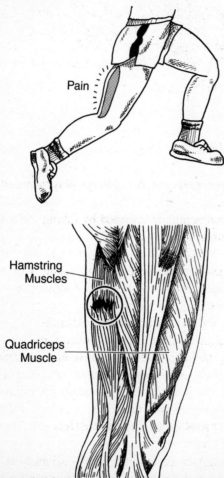

Runner's Hamstring

Massage treatment commences after any swelling has subsided and involves treating the area above the site of the injury and then below the injury. Gradually the injury will improve and after a few sessions the therapist will be able to massage on the top of the damaged muscle fibres.

A typical hamstring strain may take between one week and a month to clear with massage therapy and, in severe cases where the muscle fibres are ripped, the injury may require several months of regular treatments to heal.

There are simple and effective means to help prevent pulling a hamstring:

- Warm up the muscles thoroughly before running by massaging a warming liniment into the muscles, stretching, followed by light exercise such as running on the spot.
- Keep a consistent training schedule so that the muscles do not have an opportunity to weaken between runs, and if your training programme is disrupted for any reason, be it illness or holiday, start training again slowly.
- At the end of the run, wind down gradually by light jogging and re-stretch the muscles.

SKIER'S KNEE

The forward squatting position of a downhill skier puts great strain on the quadriceps (thigh muscles) and the tendons running through the knee joint. Consequently many skiers experience pain in and around the knees. A sudden impact of a fall can wrench the knee joint, damage the ligament tissues and tear the cartilage.

In particularly severe cases the muscles or tendons in and around the knee joint can tear and this usually requires surgery followed by regular massage treatments and remedial exer-

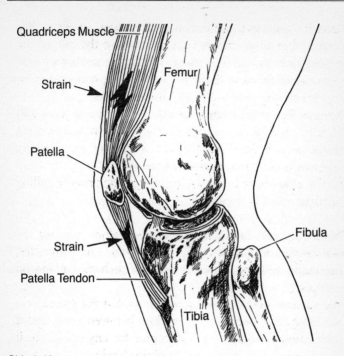

Quadriceps Muscle

Strain

Femur

Patella

Strain

Fibula

Patella Tendon

Tibia

Skier's Knee

cises. Some of the worst injuries can take over a year to recover and often require surgery.

Medical help should be sought for any large swelling to check for bone displacement or breakage and an ice pack placed on the swollen knee for 10–15 minutes every four hours. In all other cases, at the first sign of soreness around the knee, it is advisable to do alternating hot and cold compresses over the sore area. The hot compress is put on for 3 minutes followed by a cold compress for one minute and this is repeated 3 times before massage is given above and below the knee concentrating on the quadriceps. This should be carried out at least twice a day and within two days the pain should have subsided. If the pain continues seek professional help as there may be more serious damage.

After having had trouble with a knee, the muscles will be a little weak and it is therefore advisable to return to skiing gradually with a light bandage support around the knee going at least a third of the way up the quadriceps. After any injury it is important not to over-exert the muscles to ensure that the muscles do not suffer further strain.

SPRAINED ANKLE

One of the most common of all sports injuries is a sprained ankle. It affects most sports men and women including runners, football players, tennis players, rugby players, and especially squash players because of the sudden, jerky movements made in a game of squash that often have a violent impact on the ankle joint.

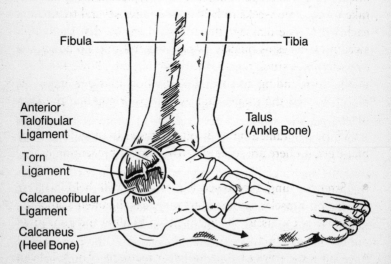

Ankle Sprain

A sprain occurs when a joint is wrenched beyond its normal range of movement damaging the surrounding tissues – ligament, tendon and muscle. The ligaments are strong fibrous tissues which encapsulate a joint to control the range of movement and help prevent it becoming displaced. Ounce for ounce, ligaments are stronger than steel and it therefore usually requires a great deal of force to damage them. Sudden impacts, an awkward twist, a fall or trip are the common causes of an ankle sprain. The ligaments are damaged by the weight of the leg's fall and are temporarily unable to hold the joint in place and the leg is then not fully supported.

The first sign of a sprain is pain, tenderness to the touch, which is swiftly followed by swelling, and there may be bruising caused by haemorrhage of the blood vessels around the joint.

It is very important that treatment is sought as soon as possible to prevent lymph fluids hardening and forming adhesions around the ligaments because these can permanently affect the joint's range of movement. A typical ankle sprain can take up to three weeks to heal and requires several treatments each week. The massage therapist will ensure that the lymph swelling reduces as quickly as possible and that no adhesions (muscle fibres stuck together with lymph) are allowed to form in the surrounding tissues. Deep friction massage improves blood flow to the tissues and also helps strengthen the ligament.

Whilst a sprained ankle is often caused by a sudden traumatic event, there are some effective ways of preventing it:

- Strengthening the lower leg muscles will help because strong muscles compensate for weak ligaments and the muscles can assist the ligaments in holding the joint in its correct position.
- Check the soles of your footwear regularly. The soles can become worn and distort your gait. Over a period of time

this causes the muscles in the lower leg to become imbalanced which gradually puts increasing strain on the ankle
joint.
- Do not do sudden jerky movements unless you are fit and
  have properly warmed up.
- Take regular hot and cold footbaths after a long game to
  help keep the tissues in the feet flexible and free from
  metabolic waste products.

RUNNER'S SHIN SPLINT

A shin splint is a condition that affects many long-distance
road runners. It manifests about 2 to 3 hours after you stop
running, creating a dull ache in the shin that is very tender to
touch. Whilst the pain is located at the front of the tibia bone
in the lower leg, it is in fact most commonly caused by torn
muscle fibres in the posterior tibial muscles which attach to the
shin bone, although on some occasions it is caused by
damaged muscle fibres in the anterior tibial muscles. The
tendons to which the muscles attach are slowly pulled away
from the bone over a period of weeks or months and then the
symptoms intensify.

The shin splint requires complete rest from running with ice
packs over the soreness to reduce the inflammation and
massage to the whole of the lower leg and foot once the
inflammation has subsided. After one week of treatment on
alternating days, the muscles may be gently stretched and
followed by strengthening exercises.

There are several preventive measures which should be
followed by all runners:

- Make sure that your running shoes are properly cushioned
  at the soles and that your foot arches are well supported. A
  shin splint is commonly preceded by a fallen arch.

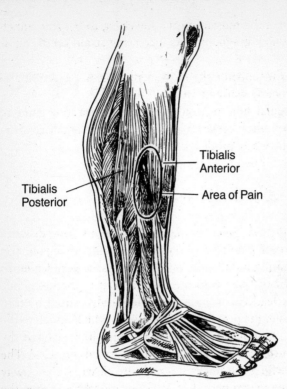

Tibialis Anterior

Area of Pain

Tibialis Posterior

Shin Splint

- Have the legs massaged regularly to prevent the gradual tearing of the muscle fibres in the lower leg.
- Warm up the muscles and stretch them before and after every run.

12
MASSAGE AND STRESS MANAGEMENT

The mind, which before massage is in a perturbed, restless, vacillating and even despondent state, becomes after massage, calm, quiet, peaceful and subdued; in fact, the wearied and worried mind has been converted into a mind restful, placid, and refreshed.

Dr Stretch Dowse, eminent Victorian physician, 1887.

WHAT IS STRESS

Stress is a subject about which the general public is becoming increasingly aware. It seems that every day a new study is reported in the press or medical journals relating stress to one disease or another. Some physicians suggest that stress may be responsible for 75 per cent of all diseases in the Western world.

Yet stress is nothing new; it has been with us since the beginning of time and is a necessary and unavoidable part of life. After all, 'stress' is actually only a word used to define physical or mental pressure or tension. You would only be free of physical stress if you were to lie still and not do any form of physical exercise. Yet, in doing so, your muscles would atrophy and waste away – if you don't use it, you lose it. And the same applies to mental stress. You only improve your memory by using your memory; you only learn by thinking. If you avoid mental stress, you must also avoid all mental activity and you will end up with a mind with the intellect of a boiled potato. So, a certain amount of stress is vital to stimulate good performance.

It is only when we take on levels of stress with which we are unable to cope that we develop stress-related problems, whether it is muscle strain from physical stress or a nervous breakdown through emotional stress. Left to accumulate, stress can cause a host of physical and emotional diseases including skin diseases (e.g., psoriasis and eczema), headaches and migraine, stomach ulcers, high blood pressure and heart-related diseases, as well as backache and muscle pain, poor eyesight and depression.

DEALING WITH PHYSICAL AND EMOTIONAL TENSION

As the world in which we live becomes increasingly stressful – both physically and emotionally – we are left with two choices: either we avoid stress or we learn how to deal with it effectively otherwise stress will overcome us. It is, of course, impossible to avoid stress, and therefore the only real solution is to find a way to manage the stresses and strains we encounter each day. One way is the use of massage.

A LEADING ROLE IN STRESS MANAGEMENT

Massage therapy offers not just effective pain relief and muscle relaxation but also a means to alleviate accumulated emotional stresses.

Sixty years ago an eminent Chicago physiologist, Dr Edmund Johnson, first recognised that anxiety was related to muscle tension. Dr Johnson noticed that people suffering from anxiety also had tense muscles. Severe anxiety tended to be accompanied by severe tension in the muscles as well. It became clear that as a person's mind became tense, so too, did his or her muscles; and conversely when the muscles became tense so too did the mind. Fortunately the reverse also holds true; if the mind is calm, the muscles tend to relax, and if the muscles are relaxed, anxiety is relieved.

The physical body and the mind's emotions are inseparable, mutually dependent, each affecting the other. Chronic physical pain such as a backache is often accompanied by depression and, similarly, anxieties can manifest themselves in a variety of physical complaints. In my experience in the practice of massage therapy, I have observed that emotional suffering is often accompanied by, and might even be influenced by, physical pain.

The most interesting example was of a middle-aged woman, Mrs M, who was married with two grown-up children who had both left home. She had been having remedial treatment for chronic pain in her upper back and shoulders. The treatment went well for several months and gradually her pain began to subside. Then one day she suddenly burst into tears during a treatment.

Using deep friction, I had finally released long-standing knotted fibres between her shoulder blades. The large knot dispersed much like a balloon popping. But I found out subsequently that the tears were not caused by any physical pain from the treatment, but rather by the sudden memory of caring for her late mother. Apparently this memory had been stored in some way, or subconsciously associated with, the muscle fibres that had knotted together.

It transpired that the chronic pains had begun when Mrs M was nursing her mother through the last days of a terminal illness, and that the painful memories had been held with the physical pain in her back. It was only when the knotted fibres in her upper back were released that she was finally able to let go of the past hurt.

In relaxing the muscles we are therefore also relaxing the mind. Such is the intricate connection of the mind with the body. It may be for this reason that massage is so successful in relieving stress. Exactly how successful massage can be was revealed in a completed study testing the effects of massage on breast cancer patients receiving radiotherapy. As you can well imagine, these women were having to deal with tremendous stress through the emotional anxiety caused by the nature of the disease on top of the physical traumas associated with radiotherapy. Those women who received back massages had less tension or tiredness and more vitality.

Anyone who has had a professional back massage will testify that it is, without doubt, one of the most effective ways of alleviating stress. A simple back massage seems to calm the body and soothe even the most troubled of minds, and enables the recipient to let go of any frustrations or anxieties at least temporarily.

REDUCING HYPERTENSION

Mr T had been one of my first clients as a massage therapist. He had been referred to me by a local acupuncturist for a relaxation back massage because he was suffering from stress and consequently from hypertension (high blood pressure). He certainly had a lot to feel stressed about, his wife had had a nervous breakdown, his father had recently died and he was having problems at work.

Mr T's blood pressure had risen to 160/110 when it really should have been in the region of 120/80. If the condition did not improve, he was told by his doctor that he would have to take drugs which could continue for the rest of his life.

I took his blood pressure before the treatment and showed it to him. It was 158/110. I then gave him a deep back massage using the 'sleep' technique to slow his breathing down and thus help his body to relax. At the end of the treatment, which was 25 minutes later, I took his blood pressure again and it showed 138/86 – a reduction of over twenty points! Mr T then returned on a regular basis and was able to control his blood pressure and thus avoided having to take medication.

THE SLEEP TECHNIQUE

A back massage is definitely one of the most relaxing massages which promotes a very deep relaxation and, in some cases, even sleep. In fact, a good massage therapist should be able to induce a deep level of relaxation using the 'sleep' technique.

The sleep technique is a method often used to help a client relax fully to relieve the effects of hypertension [high blood pressure], tension headaches and migraine. It is usually done by massaging the client's back, but it can also be done quite effectively by massaging only the neck and shoulders.

The therapist begins a normal back massage using slow, rhythmic strokes using the palmar surfaces of both hands and then gradually changes the rhythm of the strokes to that of the client's breathing pattern. After a few minutes the therapist slows the rhythm of the massage strokes and this has the effect of encouraging the client subconsciously to slow down his or her breathing to the same rhythm. One patient I saw had been unable to sleep without sleeping tablets for over 20 years, yet with the help of relaxing herbal extracts and a twice weekly relaxation massage, he was able to sleep soundly without the drugs after only eight weeks of treatment. As the weeks passed he also felt able to cut down the anti-depressant medications he had been prescribed and, with the agreement of his doctor, he came off the medications altogether two months later.

HOW MASSAGE CAN HELP TO MANAGE STRESS IN THE WORKPLACE

Stress is now being treated at the very place where it builds up worst – the workplace. Massage is so effective in managing stress that it is fast becoming a leading method of stress management in commerce and industry. In the USA there are over 4000 massage therapists who specialise in 'on-site' massage working in the offices of companies and giving relaxation massage to executives and employees. H J Heinz is one of a growing number of reputable high profile companies using 'on-site' massage therapists. At the company's world headquarters in Pittsburgh, USA, 'on-site' massage was first adopted in 1987 and massage made available to all employees during their twenty-minute coffee breaks. Fifteen-minute massages are given to each client's head, neck and shoulders – the areas where most people carry the bulk of their tensions.

According to Gene Arbetter, spokesman for the American Massage Therapy Association in Chicago, 'The boom in OSM [on-site massage] has revolutionised workplace health, not just because employees like it. When a company buys OSM, it pays for itself: employees don't need as many sick or "mental health" days if they have an outlet for tension at work.'

In the UK 'on-site' massage is also becoming increasingly popular. The TSB Trust Company in Leeds was one of the first to adopt it with over 50 per cent of its work force taking advantage of the service. Ronnie Campbell, the regional sales manager, said, 'All the staff being treated regularly feel much more relaxed. The massage has been very therapeutic and has dispersed the frequent neck strains and headaches. There is no doubt the massage has had a cumulative benefit, resulting in employees feeling less lethargic and more full of energy.'

Massage has proven to be such an effective form of stress management that even the UK police force have begun to co-opt the services of massage therapists to help relieve the daily stresses undergone by police officers. Chief Superintendent Peter Twist initiated the project at Limehouse police station in the East End of London in 1989 and the scheme was so well received that another police station in Chelmsford, Essex is planning to follow suit. 'Unless you're very honest and open,' said the Superintendent, 'you don't recognise you're suffering from stress. Most of us deal with it by going down to the pub, drinking three or four pints and having a night on the town; I'm saying, get on the massage table instead.'

So, although stress can affect us in many different areas of our lives, massage is a natural and extremely efficient physical medicine in the treatment of stress-related disorders, and is now taking a leading role in the development of stress management techniques in medical centres, hospitals, in the workplace and in the home.

RECOMMENDED READING

Athletic Massage by Rich Phaigh & Paul Perry, Simon & Schuster (1984).

Back to Eden by Jethro Kloss, Back to Eden Publishing Co (1939).

Chinese Massage Therapy by Lee Whincup, Routledge & Kegan Paul Ltd (1983).

The Complete Book of Massage by Clare Maxwell-Hudson, Dorling Kindersley Publishers Ltd (1988).

The Complete Guide to Stress Management by Dr Chandra Patel, Optima (1989).

Massage – Principles and Techniques by G. Beard & E. Wood, Saunders (1964).

Reflex Zone Therapy by Hanne Marquardt, Thorsens (1983).

USEFUL ADDRESSES

U.K.
London College of
   Aromatherapy,
Swanfleet Centre,
93 Fortress Road,
London NW5 1AG.

The Institute of Complementary
   Medicine,
21 Portland Place,
London W1N 3AF.

College of Holistic Medicine,
4 Craigpark,
Glasgow G31 2NA.

The Northern Institute of
   Massage,
100 Waterloo Road,
Blackpool FY4 1AW.

International College of Oriental
   Medicine,
Green Hedges House,
Green Hedges Avenue,
East Grinstead,
Sussex RH19 1DZ.

The London & Counties Society
   of Physiologists,
330 Lytham Road,
Blackpool, Lancs FY4 1DW.

Canada
Ontario Massage Therapy
   Association
456 Danforth Avenue,
Toronto, Ontario M4K 1P4.

Northern Institute of Massage,
Box No 37, Clyde,
Alberta, T0G 0P0.

Western College of Remedial
   Massage Therapies,
Box No 33004, Regina,
Saskatchewan S4S 7X2.

U.S.A.
The American Massage Therapy
   Association,
Chicago.

INDEX